SO WHAT THE F*** SHOULD I EAT?

The fat loss plan that cuts through the confusion - and delivers!

Fiona Kirk

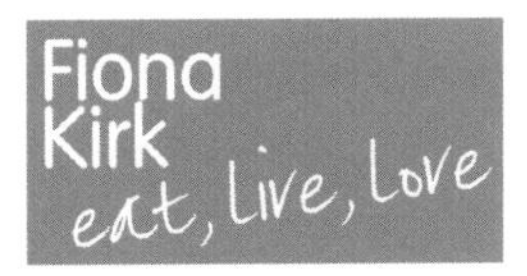

For more information visit
www.fionakirk.com

Painless Publishing

Published in the UK 2010 by **Painless Publishing**
www.painlesspublishing.com

Note to readers

If you are pregnant, breastfeeding, on regular medication, have concerns about your health or are under the age of 16 you should consult your doctor or health practitioner before embarking on any new eating and/or exercise programme. Every effort has been made to present the information in this book in a clear, complete and accurate manner, however not every situation can be anticipated and the information in this book cannot take the place of a medical analysis of individual health needs. The author and Painless Publishing hereby disclaim any and all liability resulting from injuries or damage caused by following any recommendations in this book.

References

All statements (other than personal views) and studies referred to throughout the book have been exhaustively researched but the author chose not to reference them throughout the text and add copious additional pages at the back of the book. Should you wish further information about any of the above, email through the author's website, www.fionakirk.com and they will be provided promptly.

Typesetting **Max Morris, Milkbar Creative / Ideas and Creations**
Cover Design **Max Morris, Milkbar Creative / Ideas and Creations**
Images **Isla Munro**
Chapter Introductions **Liam Smith**

225pp

ISBN 978 0 9566115 0 5

About Me

This book is about you, not about me but perhaps a few revelations about how I came to write it may inspire you!

I was a skinny kid and possibly due to the fact that I was always far too busy to get my eight hours plus per night (much to my parents' frustration), I failed to reach much over five feet tall. I wasn't a particularly picky eater but then, when I was growing up food was a great deal plainer and choice a lot more limited than it is now - Scotch Broth, cold meat and chips on Monday, macaroni cheese on Tuesday, mince and tatties on Wednesday, fish in breadcrumbs on Thursday , roast chicken for Sunday lunch etc. And, if you didn't finish your greens you rarely got pudding.

My mum was, and still is a great baker so there was always a couple of pancakes, a chocolate crispy or a slice of gingerbread with a generous slathering of cold butter when we came home from school and we were encouraged to help with the baking which invariably meant we were allowed to lick the bowl. How things have changed!

When I reached puberty, despite being very sporty I started to thicken around the middle - could it possibly have been anything to do with the pancakes? Around the age of 15, lots of my friends were going on diets so I followed suit. We tried everything from disgusting herbal concoctions to endless days of starvation. We usually lost weight but of course we couldn't keep it up for long and hit the cream buns at break time with a passion!

I suppose you could say that I learned early on that most diets don't work but, like many that never held me back from leaping into the unknown - the promise was always tantalising. But I never became a yo-yo or serial dieter. Why? Because I love food! I love eating it, I love reading about it, I love planning, shopping, preparing and cooking for eating extravaganzas with friends and family, I am addicted to Jamie, Gordon, Nigel, Delia, Masterchef, Saturday Kitchen and the rest and I love eating out, experimenting with cuisines from Turkey to Thailand and everywhere in between.

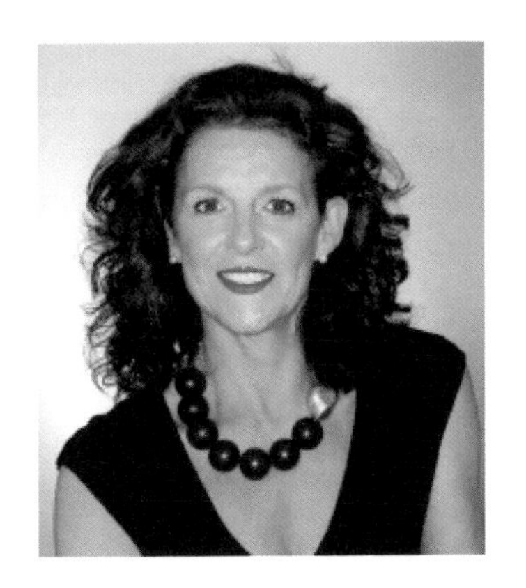

But, back to my mum. Her interest in cooking, baking and entertaining on a scale that I will never be able to compete with was, and still is a huge influence.

She wanted to know more and experimented with recipes from some of the greats during the 70's and 80's including Arabella Boxer, the *Galloping Gourmet,* Graham Kerr, the Roux Brothers, Antonio Carluccio and Prue Leith and I continue to call her on a regular basis with culinary enquiries when a dish isn't coming together.

So, how did I eventually halt the ever-thickening middle? Firstly, I recognised that a size 14 is not a good look for someone who is barely over five feet tall and secondly, I had a very early menopause. Everything I read about *the change of life* mentioned probable weight gain which meant I was looking at a possible size 16 or 18 if I didn't take drastic action. HRT was not an option as research was flagging up an increased risk of breast cancer if used long-term so I started looking at complimentary medical tactics. Eureka! I discovered that what, when and how I eat might have an influence not only on balancing my now-less-than-optimally-performing sex hormones but also on why the fat was happily storing itself around my waistline. I needed to know more so I made the somewhat irrational decision at 40-something to enrol as a student at The Institute for Optimum Nutrition in London and spent the next 4 years learning a new trade.

It was long, it was hard, it was near-impossible sometimes to juggle work commitments, domestic arrangements, monthly tutorials in London and a hefty load of homework but boy did I learn a lot. I have to point out that it was a good few years after I qualified before I started to get rid of the fat around my middle. Why? Because it took years of consultation with hundreds of clients before I realised that our personal weight loss goals can only be achieved when we address our own priorities, our own eating patterns, our own circumstances and our own crazy indulgences.

That's why I wrote this book. Fad diets work for some, prescriptive diets work for others, super-sensible eating plans work for the disciplined amongst us, frantic exercise programmes work for few. It is only when we find the diet that fits our life and includes the foods that make us feel good and satisfy our needs that we can lose the *love handles* or the *man boobs* and feel good - my aim is to cut through some of the confusion that is coming at you from all sides and spare you the years of study that got me, ultimately to a heathy and fit size 10.

And I still *eat*, *live* and *love* food - particularly pancakes!

And Another Thing...

Whilst I have endeavoured to make this book an easy read, it is impossible to pass on some of the important messages without resorting to the use of technical nutritional terms on occasion. There is a glossary at the back of the book which I hope explains all - refer to it whenever you come across any words/principles that require further explanation and if you want more information, email me through my website **www.fionakirk.com**. The aim is to cut through the confusion not add to it!

Table of Contents

PART TWO: What You Need to Know to Cut through the Confusion

PART THREE:
How to be Radical, Reckless or Dedicated to a Plan

Introduction

How do you usually approach a diet?

It's Monday morning and the start of another week and this is going to be *the first day of the rest of your life*. This time you are determined. You are going to lose weight and keep it off. You are going to follow the eating, drinking and exercise recommendations and failure is not an option. It's going to mean a lot of change but you know that change is required. No more cheating, quitting or excuses – this is *the one*, the way forward. You may not be familiar with some of the recommended foods or eating practices involved but you will learn to love them as you learn to love watching the pounds melt away. Sound familiar?

So, why shouldn't they melt away?

Well, one reason they may not shift is if you don't know where they came from. Sounds simple because it is! If you are carting excess pounds of flesh around because you always choose the cheeseburger over the seasonal salad or the fizzy *pop* over the fizzy water or the deep fried cod over the steamed fish you already know that this kind of *road accident* of a diet needs some improvement. All you have to do is substitute the *good* for the *bad*, cut back on the portions, get to the gym a bit more regularly and the flab should start to shift. Hard work but reasonably straightforward and with a little guidance and a lot of support can be done.

But, what if you are already trying your damnedest to get *5-a-Day* into your life, regularly say no to unhealthy options, exercise a few times a week, cook fresh as often as possible and still can't lose weight? Not so straightforward. You don't know where the flab came from or indeed why it won't budge.

Either way, there's a mountain to climb and unless you have the kit it can be an uphill struggle. But in no way is it insurmountable!

So how can you make it work? By turning your diet on its head and making a few crazy decisions. Probably everything you have ever heard or read about losing weight concentrates on adopting some sort of routine. But a routine that works for whom? Often someone else, usually not you! On one hand there are the wacky programmes that concentrate on removing all sorts of things from your life for a time (we're talking deprivation here), on the other hand there are the *experts* who champion a balance of essential nutrients which form the basis of a healthy diet which once embraced will set you up for a lifetime of weight maintenance and vitality (we're talking sensible here, but often dull and repetitive). The reason you have bought (or are about to buy) this book is possibly because you have tried both methods and they haven't worked.

Fancy trying an altogether more exciting and adventurous route? Read on. If you truly want to lose weight you have to make the decisions that work for you, not the decisions others make for you. Safe and sensible decisions are often boring, predictable and take you nowhere new. Unsafe and reckless decisions cause you to think and respond in a way you may not have thought about previously and may help you achieve what you want and perhaps even take you to a place you have only dreamt of.

Don't just follow the crowd, there's no fun in that. Take the rebellious or outrageous route and find what works for you. Have the courage to discover what you may be missing out on and when it comes to weight loss there are rarely wrong or reckless decisions – just misguided caution that prompts you to play safe.

The aim of this book is to delve into why there is so much confusion about diet and why shifting fat for good has become so complicated that many ultimately decide just to get used to a bigger waistline and shop accordingly. My goal is to cut through the confusion and give you what you want.

You want to burn fat, not store it!

So here goes

Part One offers some debate on what's on offer and exposes some of the nonsensical, unworkable advice that forms a major part of the confusion, part two provides the stuff you need to know to boost your resolve, increase your understanding and help you make the decisions that are going to work for you and part three gives you the opportunity to be radical, reckless or dedicated to a plan.

Success could be around the corner when you put your priorities first and devise a diet that fits in with your life, your timetable, your tastes and yes, your indulgences.

Part 1. Chapter One

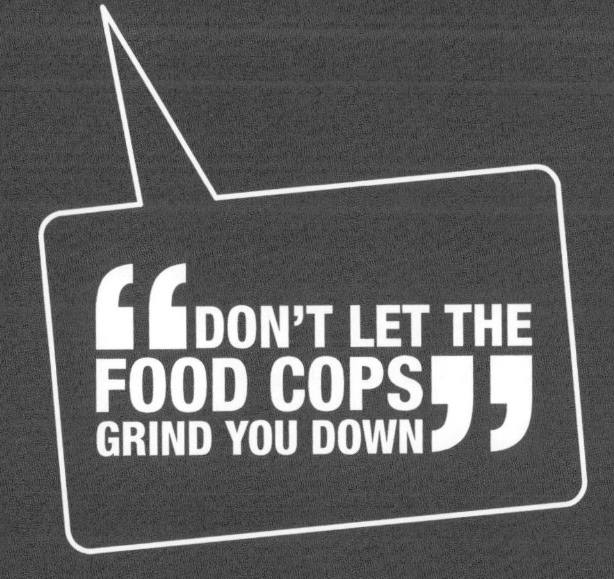

Put the food down and walk slowly forward with your mouth shut and nobody gets hurt!

This chapter looks at why scare tactics, rebukes and government directives are unlikely to result in people giving up the foods they love and adopt a healthier diet and suggests that there may be altogether more intelligent and creative ways to encourage us to look our dietary demons in the eye and lose fat for good.

Confused?

Put the food DOWN and walk slowly forward with your mouth shut and nobody gets hurt! This says it all really. The weekly shop is stressful enough as we try to stock the fridge, keep in budget and suit everybody's tastes. Healthy options abound but it's hard to make the right decisions 100% of the time when there is so much choice and confusion reigns supreme. If there's one thing we don't need, it's the *food police*. Even if they are not actually in the aisles yet, we know they are out there waiting to pounce on our shopping trolleys and serve us with a food ASBO!

So What Sucks?

Our Diet is Killing us

Or so the nutritional scaremongers would have us believe. Oh, to open the daily newspaper and learn that at least some of our food choices merit a gold star. Sadly, many people appear to be getting it more wrong than right and are staring cancer, heart problems, diabetes and a host of degenerative diseases in the face.

The *worthies* are eager to remind us that charred and barbecued foods create known carcinogens - even burnt toast is suspect, sugar kills our sex life, heavily salted, smoked and pickled foods lead to higher rates of stomach cancer, chips and snack foods contain fats that block arteries leading to heart disease and stroke, excess alcohol increases the risk of breast, larynx, oesophageal and mouth cancer, farmed fish contain liver-damaging toxins, the sodium nitrate in hot dogs are believed to hasten pancreatic cancer, *acrylamide* found in many baked goods is a human carcinogen-suspect, chemicals in food packaging pose threats and the debate over the dangers of *aspartame* in diet drinks rages on.

We're all doomed unless we sharpen up!

Tough talk has become the new route to convincing us to ditch our poor eating habits and adopt a better diet. A table laden with the weekly food intake of a few unsuspecting overweight volunteers followed by a series of rebukes about how the bulk of these foods are shortening their lives has become a popular media method of forcing people to look their dietary demons in the eye and prompt a u-turn. Scare tactics may work for some but for many alarm bells ring creating fear and doubt about every food decision. Hardly the road to enlightenment.

Are We Really That Stupid?

Some *experts* suggest that we are making food decisions based on a degree of ignorance. We have simply lost or perhaps never had the ability to determine between foods that improve our chance of a long and healthy life and those that are either questionable or downright detrimental. We prefer to remain blissfully unaware of the long term health implications of a diet centred round fast, junk and processed foods and dietetic and nutritional *gods* are needed to help us see the error of our ways. Words like reduce, resist, restrict and avoid invade every paragraph of the mantra from the diet messiahs and their message is clear – we need help and they are here to give it.

I believe that most people are aware that 'Big Macs', 'Stuffed Crust' Pizzas, Fish Suppers, Donner Kebabs and cans of Coca Cola will never make it onto the list of foods recommended for good health and that fruits, vegetables, whole grains, beans, lentils, nuts, seeds and water will always get top grades but continual reminders about how appalling our eating habits have become are not enough to encourage us to let go of our favourites. I often ask clients and audiences which teachers, tutors or bosses help them achieve their ambitions and most agree that it is those who invite discussion and debate whilst providing encouragement and guidance that inspire them. Few praise the individuals who simply tell them what to do with little time for their views or concerns. Surely people would be more likely to consider dietary improvements if a similar strategy were employed?

There are also many who point out that some food manufacturers are more interested in pleasing shareholders than looking after long-term health needs. Until demand for sugary, salty, fatty, junk and fast foods dries up manufacturers will continue to produce them and profit from our unhealthy choices. The consumer dictates the market so the consumer is, in part to blame. Yet another responsibility we have to shoulder.

Could it be that opting for the 'Big Mac' and other fast food choices over the adzuki bean stew and healthier options is not so much an ignorant choice, more a quick, convenient and affordable choice that people make because time and money are short? Supermarkets give us endless opportunities to save pounds on our weekly shop but it probably has not escaped your attention that...

***Buy one get one free* stickers on multi-packs of processed foods far outweigh those on packs of broccoli!**

Obesity Tax

Some health campaigners are in favour of introducing a 'fat tax' into the UK to tackle the obesity epidemic. There are different forms such a tax could take. One proposal is to tax foods that contain too much fat or salt or to target sugary snacks and fizzy drinks, another is to charge VAT on foods that are currently zero rated but are believed to be contributing to the problem. Revenue from these taxes would be used to finance subsidies for healthy foods or exercise equipment in schools, colleges and the workplace and fund advertising campaigns encouraging healthy eating.

The rationale behind these proposals is that if we have to pay more for junk food we will buy less of it. The government already uses tax to influence behaviour with high taxes on cigarettes, alcohol and petrol so why not food? Simplistic or what? The globally increasing waistline won't be halted merely by hitting people where it hurts – their wallets. There are many underlying reasons why some people gain weight year on year whilst others don't. Believing that obesity statistics can be reduced and consumer behaviour changed without looking at the whole picture has to be *big brother* at his ridiculous best and may start a revolution. Bring it on!

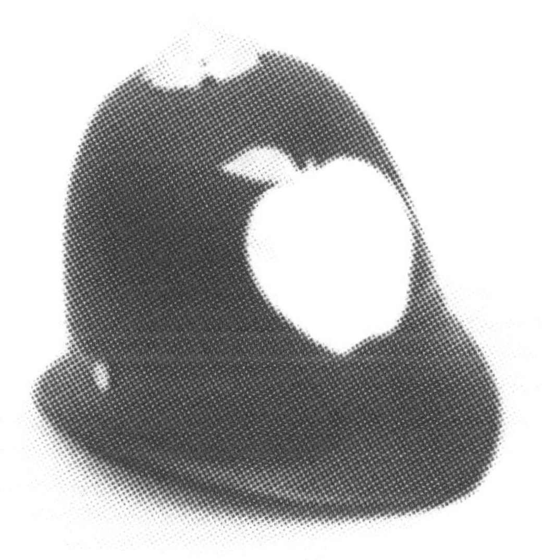

So What's Sound?

Progress Causes Weight Gain

Some argue that our DNA has barely changed since man first evolved and that we are genetically unable to adapt to the modern diet. Our ancient genes are routinely exposed to unfamiliar food molecules causing confusion within body cells, altering the way they behave and triggering inflammation. Weight gain and inflammation are strongly linked. There are a number of fundamental changes that have taken place in food processing that some believe to be at the root of the problem.

Refined cereal grains form a large part of many diets, particularly foods made with white flour (bread, rolls, pasta, cakes, biscuits, snacks, pies, tarts etc.)

and white rice. Grains were rare in our pre-agricultural diet and those that were available were unrefined. The hefty load of refined grains we now consume not only means we are losing out on vitamins, minerals and fibre but also upsetting the ratio of carbohydrates, proteins and fats required in a balanced diet. Vitamins, minerals, fibre and a balance of the three major food groups are essential for fat loss. See chapter 6, *A Little Knowledge is not a Dangerous Thing* for more information on why a good mix of the above is so important.

The domestication of animals, which introduced **dairy foods and cultivated meats** (again, non-existent items in our pre-agricultural diet) changed the composition of our fat intake by adding large amounts of saturated fats to our diet whilst seriously reducing essential fats.

Fats are important for fat loss - some help, others don't.

The third and some think worst change is our love affair with **sugar**. Sugar was also rare in the hunter-gatherer diet – just honey occasionally and the sugars in seasonal fruits. Refined sugar and all the high-fructose syrups that are now added to our foods are playing havoc with our insulin delivery mechanism and increasing the likelihood of both weight gain and type 2 diabetes on a global scale. When the overload of glucose derived from these types of sugars is not required to create energy it is quickly dumped into fat stores where it remains until it is forced into action.

The hunter-gatherer rarely used **salt.** It wasn't mined and it was not added to food. Water, seaweed, meat, fish and vegetation provided natural sources of sodium which is vital for blood pressure maintenance and the functioning of nerves and muscles. The amount of salt in our diet now has played a mean trick by upsetting the balance of sodium to potassium in body cells. Too many processed foods and too few fruits and vegetables means too much sodium and not enough potassium and an increased risk of high blood pressure. Not a problem our ancestors had to address. A twenty year experiment in Finland during the 1970's and 80's saw a large proportion of the nation switching from sodium-rich table salt to a mixed potassium and magnesium-rich salt. Blood pressure levels and the incidence of heart attacks and strokes fell dramatically (by an average of 60%). Some of the larger supermarkets stock *Solo Sea Salt*, usually in the 'speciality' section which is low in sodium and high in potassium and magnesium. If you use salt in cooking try to make the switch and reduce the risks.

Technology has led to the development of **processed vegetable oils** which are often high in hydrogenated and semi hydrogenated fats and are even worse for our health than over-consumption of saturated fats. But they are everywhere. They make foods more palatable, spreadable and moreish and extend the shelf life of a great many products – a dream come true for food manufacturers but difficult for the body to metabolise and tragically nutrient-poor. They are itemised on food labels so avoid products containing them when you can.

Fibre averaged about 100 grams per day in the hunter-gatherer diet and came almost exclusively from roots, fruits, nuts, seeds and vegetation. Processing strips foods of their fibre making them easier to chew and quick to digest which is why they are popular. But we need fibre - to clean our genetically-programmed ancient gut, remove toxins and promote fat loss. Now we are lucky to get an average of 20 grams per day and from a very narrow range of sources.

There is also huge concern about the **loss of micronutrients** in the soil used for mass food production. Are we are getting the full complement of nutrients required to meet our energy requirements, fight off disease and keep us in the fat burning *zone* or should we be supplementing our diet? This subject attracts more argument than perhaps any other in the nutritional arena. After years of helping people to shed fat and feel great I have concluded that many find sticking to a supplement regime almost as hard if not harder than sticking to a diet regime. Plus, good quality supplements are expensive so when we don't see quick results we stop. My advice is always the same.

Start by gradually improving your diet but if you suspect that your lifestyle and food choices are preventing you from reaching your daily nutritional requirements consider supplementation. Resist the temptation to self medicate as this route can be costly and may not meet your needs.

If you can, make an appointment with a nutritional therapist who will analyse your health status and diet and after discussion may recommend specific nutrients to make up for any deficiencies. One consultation could save a fortune in the long run.

Our over-consumption of **foods that produce acidity** within the body prompting inflammation and an increased risk of disease is another key issue. As with every aspect of human biochemistry, homeostasis (balance) is vital. A diet overloaded with sugary, salty and fatty foods producing acidity and light on fruits, vegetables and essential fats which counteract the acidity weakens our immune system and impairs our resistance to all manner of viral and bacterial threats. The common cold or a bout of mild food poisoning are inconvenient and debilitating but most of us recover fairly quickly. However, some of the recent viruses that have crossed continents because of the growth in international travel demand a strong immune system if we are to avoid them (the recent swine flu epidemic is an example). In essence, we are simply not consuming sufficient alkaline-forming foods to achieve a healthy acid:alkaline balance. Where there is imbalance and inflammation there is unlikely to be fat loss.

So the dictum is lots of whole grains, watch dairy produce, fear cultivated meat, don't even think about sugar, bin the salt, bypass processed food shelves and eat foods the way nature intended. It all makes sense but possibly leaves many of us feeling more than a little inadequate when we fail to reach many or any of these targets.

So What Rocks?

Take a Risk or Two!

Life is risky. Every action holds the potential for success or failure. Many of us are scared of taking any kind of risk that moves us out of our comfort zone and prefer to follow the pack. Others blindly throw caution to the wind with little regard to the consequences. A calculated risk however is one that has been given careful thought, one where we have weighed up and examined the risks and rewards and the potential upside outweighs the potential downside. In other words, a risk worth taking. Changing our eating habits and adopting a new approach to how we nourish our bodies is a risky business and can present all manner of daily challenges that can take us well outside our comfort zone but the rewards can be great and the feeling of achievement even greater.

Make a List or Two

Get a large piece of paper and write down all the foods and drinks you love. Put down as much information as you can then take another piece of paper and try to work out why you love them. Is it the look, smell, taste, sound or just the thought? Have you enjoyed them since childhood and eat them out of habit or are some of them connected to specific activities (popcorn at the movies, fry-ups on a Sunday morning etc?)

Are some of them associated with comfort? When you are down or tired or cold or stressed or chasing your tail do you invariably head for the same old food solutions? When you are out do you generally go to the same bars, cafes and restaurants and have your familiar favourites? Do you sometimes struggle to say no for fear of upsetting people or drawing attention to the fact that you are *on* a diet? Does your shopping list change little from week to week and if so why? Are you always short of time or is it just easier and cheaper to churn out the same old meals?

When you weigh up and examine the pros and cons of the food choices you make currently and determine why some of them may be thwarting your desire for better health, increased fitness or fat loss you can take calculated risks and map a route to success.

This little exercise can take a bit of time but if you seriously want the fat to budge it can be a real winner. What many people find is that there is a lot less variety in their diet than they thought and variety is the key when it comes to fat loss. Fat cells won't be goaded into releasing their stored energy and shrink if the body doesn't get the full spectrum of macronutrients (carbohydrates, protein and fats) and micronutrients (vitamins, minerals and accessory nutrients). Permanent fat loss can only be achieved when all the tools are to hand and work together.

Once you have completed your *love* list, do the same with the foods and drinks you hate. This can be very revealing. Reasons given for hating certain foods often include such words as boring, difficult, tasteless, unappetising, gross, unexciting, unappealing and sometimes just too damned healthy. Looking over your *hate* list and recognising that foods that should ideally be included in a healthy diet feature heavily can be dispiriting but learning to love some of them as you love watching the pounds of fat melt away is easier than you might think. Read on.

Eat More

The *calorie myth* has been around for so long that it is almost impossible to avoid. But it can be one of biggest stumbling blocks when it comes to permanent fat loss. The basic principle is that if we take in fewer calories than we expend we will lose weight. The UK government 'watchdog', The Food Standards Authority and many other health and weight loss *experts* advise that "to lose 1lb of fat you need to either reduce your calorie intake by 3500kcals per week or increase your exercise levels, preferably both". Here's how it is supposed to work. If a woman currently weighs 120lbs (around eight and a half stones) and regularly consumes around 2500kcals per day which is, dependent on her age, height and level of physical activity around 500kcals more than the recommended requirement and reduces her intake by 500kcals per day (that's a large bag of kettle chips, a cheese and tomato pizza or a portion of lasagne) she will lose one to two pounds of weight every seven days. If she continues this for a year she should be 52lbs lighter which would make her just under 5 stones and before the second year is out she will have disappeared – and she hasn't even put her trainers on!

But of course she won't disappear because her body will compensate and turn down the rate at which her food is metabolised, burning calories at a slower rate and storing life-preserving energy as fat. Why and how this happens is discussed in chapter 5, *Rule Number One – There are No Rules*.

If the *calories in versus calories out* theory is the definitive route to weight loss why are we gaining weight globally despite the fact that many are following this advice? Why have levels of obesity tripled since 1980 in the UK and year on year we sit way too comfortably amongst the top six nations whose waistbands grow ever larger? Why, despite the huge increase in sales of low calorie and low fat products are sales of size 16+ clothes keeping pace?

Why, despite the huge increase in sales of low calorie and low fat products are sales of size 16+ clothes keeping pace?

Calories are a useful yardstick to measure the *quantity* of calories in food but tell us little about the *quality*. The number of calories a person needs to consume daily for fat loss depends on various factors including age, sex, current health status, level and type of daily exercise, amount of muscle and percentage of body fat. In order to get nourishment from food the body works to a basic set of rules. For example, bread, pasta, rice and cereals are processed one way, burgers, chicken and fish another, fats and oils yet another. As far as the body is concerned the overriding rule is always the same – gain the maximum possible nourishment from everything consumed and make the best use of it to create energy, repair, rebuild and protect body cells, feed the brain, bones and muscles and keep defences strong. It is a very sophisticated machine but unlike a machine it doesn't stop working when the instructions aren't followed precisely. It has the ability to adapt to a host of different circumstances which are as individual as we are.

Eating too much, consuming too many calories whilst doing little or no exercise results in weight gain over time for most people, just as eating too little and consuming too few calories whilst exercising ferociously results in weight loss more often than not. Both routes present a major challenge to the body long term as it struggles to cope and both routes carry health risks. Great foods that provide great nourishment allow the body to do the job it was designed for and it is short-sighted to expect it to complete its many tasks on a daily basis if it is deficient in energy-rich quality calories.

Quality v Quantity

A ready meal of chicken tikka masala with pilau rice from the supermarket provides around 450kcals per portion, so do two Cadbury's Crème Eggs. A large homemade salad with grilled chicken, lettuce, tomato, cucumber, sun-dried tomatoes, grilled peppers, courgettes, peas, sweetcorn, feta cheese and pine nuts dressed with olive oil and lemon juice provides around 550kcals but gives the body a wealth of nutrients. And let's say any one of these choices were repeated four times a day. Four chicken tikka masala with pilau rice or eight Cadbury's Crème Eggs = 1800kcals, four salads = 2000kcals but which provides the best nourishment and is most likely to promote fat loss? The salad of course. Yes, it has the highest calorie count but it contains a fabulous combination of nutrients and quality calories. The Cadburys Crème Egg don't even come close and the chicken tikka masala, whilst providing some useful nutrients can't really compete.

Another misplaced myth is that people who are seriously overweight or clinically obese simply eat too much and don't take enough exercise. Weight loss studies involving people of both sexes with a body mass index (BMI) which puts them in the overweight/obese category show that many are eating way below their recommended daily calorie intake but don't lose weight which further questions the *calories in versus calories out* theory. There are, of course genetic, health and behavioural reasons why serious weight gain occurs and long term weight loss doesn't - these can only be identified and treated with the help of professionals. Understanding where to find the quality calories that meet our personal energy requirements is the first step. Getting them in balance is the second. It is vital to recognise that for some this may involve eating more, for others less. Personal nutritional requirements must be met to encourage fat burning.

Continual calorie counting may well be the reason many people are still looking for a way to lose fat for good.

Bin the Scales

A lean, fit body is a body with plenty of working muscle. Muscle is active and requires a lot of energy from food. Muscle is also denser than body fat so takes up less room pound for pound. If you lose two pounds of fat while gaining two pounds of muscle body weight won't change but body shape will – for the better, so what you actually weigh is in some instances immaterial. Professional sportsmen and women, soldiers in the armed forces, bodybuilders etc who have plenty of muscle and little body fat generally weigh more than their *couch potato* counterparts but their bodies look a great deal fitter and healthier despite the fact that their weight puts many of them in the overweight category if their BMI is used as a benchmark. More on the confusion surrounding BMI later. You need only look in the mirror or put on your tightest jeans to see that fat cells are shrinking nicely. Details of the *Waistband Method* and how to keep a check on weekly fat loss are covered in chapter 13, *The Fat Loss Plan of Action*.

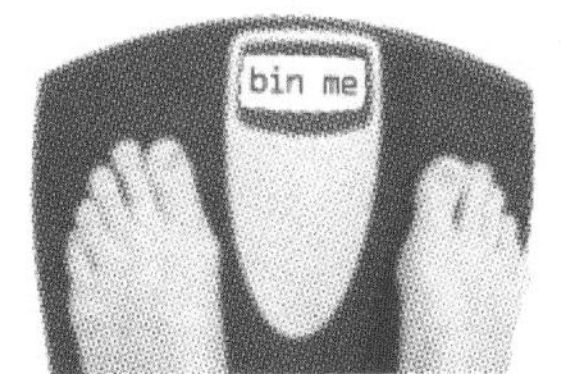

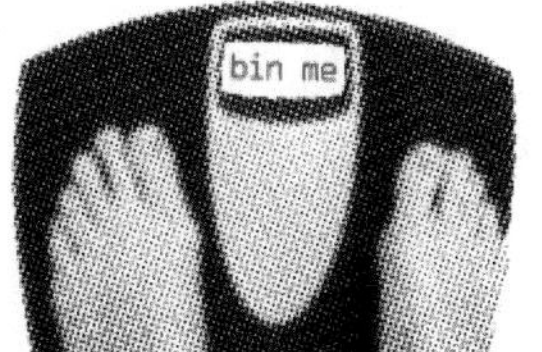

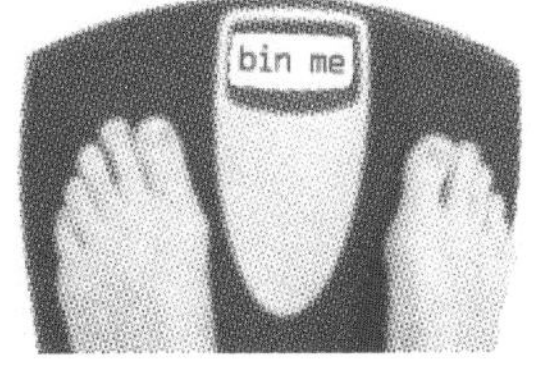

Part 1. Chapter Two

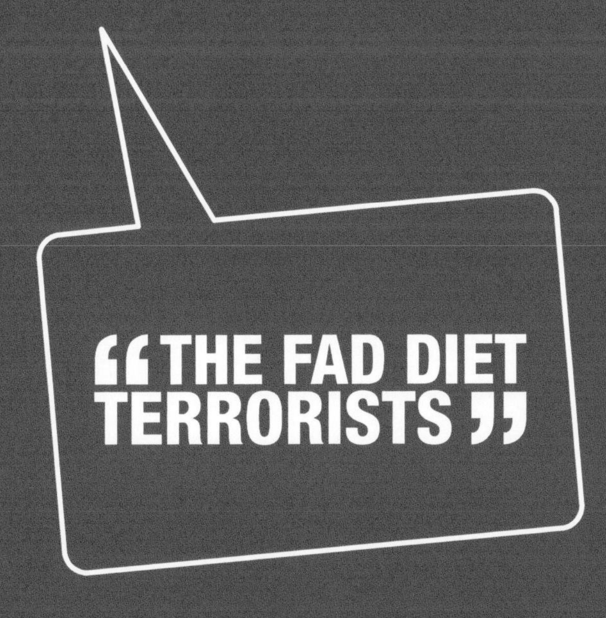

Whether it's points or grams or blueberries or calories, counting = hassle!

This chapter looks at why diets don't always fail despite the negative press many receive. A few of the most popular diets are discussed with a few cautionary notes on why many are best left on the bookshelf. But it's not all doom and gloom. There are nuggets of gold to be found when you know where to look which can be used to help build a personal *Fat Loss Plan* that works.

Confused?

Diets don't work. Statistics show that around **90% of dieters regain the weight they lost within 18 months** so why waste time and money – we are cursed from the start. *Fad* diets come in for the greatest criticism and are regarded as the villains when it comes to our increasing waistlines. Other than their creators and promoters it is difficult to find anyone who has a good word to say about them.

Here are a few of the negatives:-

- They cause excess weight gain when we quit.
- They have detrimental effects on our metabolism.
- They result in nutritional deficiencies.
- They are unrealistic and impossible to stick to in the long term.
- They are backed by testimonials that can't be scrutinised.
- They may result in serious health problems.
- They produce weight loss only by reducing calorie intake.
- They are promoted using bogus science or nutritional advice.

But what about the 10% of dieters who don't fail?

Do they all see the light, adopt a healthy lifestyle, learn to say no to *Krispy Kremes* and change their eating habits for life? What have successful dieters discovered that the rest of us may have missed? In essence, they have discovered that a diet that works for them fits their eating patterns, lifestyle, tastes and energy requirements; a diet they can live with and enjoy. But does it happen overnight? Rarely. Trial and error are usually involved. The successful dieter is able to recognise the unworkable aspects of a programme and concentrate on the recommendations that are easily slotted into their daily life.

So where do we start and who do we believe?

So What Sucks?

Cynics

That growing band who suggest that diets are a marketing ploy aimed at duping the dieter whilst boosting sales of books, foods and supplements. Difficult to believe in all cases. Many are designed by professionals who want to help and motivate people to improve their health and lose weight. Writing a diet book or creating a weight loss website involves an investment of time and more often than not, money. Publication is usually followed by a waiting period while the media and the *experts* decide whether to spin it, endorse it or bin it then we, the discerning consumers choose to adopt it or ignore it. Desperation to lose a few pounds does not guarantee dieters are going to buy into every new approach. If that were the case, most diets would succeed commercially and they don't. For every one that creates a stir and becomes a *fad* there are thousands that sit on the bookshelves gathering dust and are never reprinted or remain largely *un-googled* before disappearing into the ether. Then it's back to the drawing board for the creator coupled with a huge dent to both self-esteem and bank balance.

Ignorance

A diet that works has to make sense to the dieter. Understanding and believing that before you start is vital. The promise of weight loss is not enough. People who make diets work, achieve their goal by doing three things. Firstly, they recognise the potential personal pitfalls of the programme – how much does it cost, will it fit in with their lifestyle, are the foods easy to find, prepare and cook, are they willing to experiment etc. Secondly, they take time to read and understand the principles behind the diet. Some are ground-breaking, some are dubious and some are downright daft so if there's any doubt leave it on the bookshelf – it's not going to work. Thirdly, they have the right attitude. They attack the programme with all the enthusiasm and positive mental attitude they can muster. Little doubts can quickly turn into big negatives and the only thing that comes crashing down is resolve, not weight.

There will never be a 'one shoe size fits all' diet. No two of us look exactly the same, have the same tastes in food, culture, fashion or partners nor do we metabolise food identically so no two of us can expect the same result from a fat loss programme. Many of us make the mistake of embarking on a diet that saw a workmate or friend steadily losing weight without considering that their lifestyle, tastes and energy requirements are a million miles away from our own. When we drop only a few pounds while they are complaining that they have to buy a new wardrobe because all their clothes are 'hanging off' we become frustrated and dispirited. It's an unfair but common occurrence.

Fat loss can be achieved when we feel good and properly nourished not hungry and miserable - when we recognise potential pitfalls and adopt a strategy to deal with them.

Ask yourself the three questions before you dive into any diet:

1. What are the potential personal pitfalls and can they be managed/overcome?
2. Do I understand and believe in the principles behind the promised weight/fat loss?
3. Do I have the right attitude to make it work – and last?

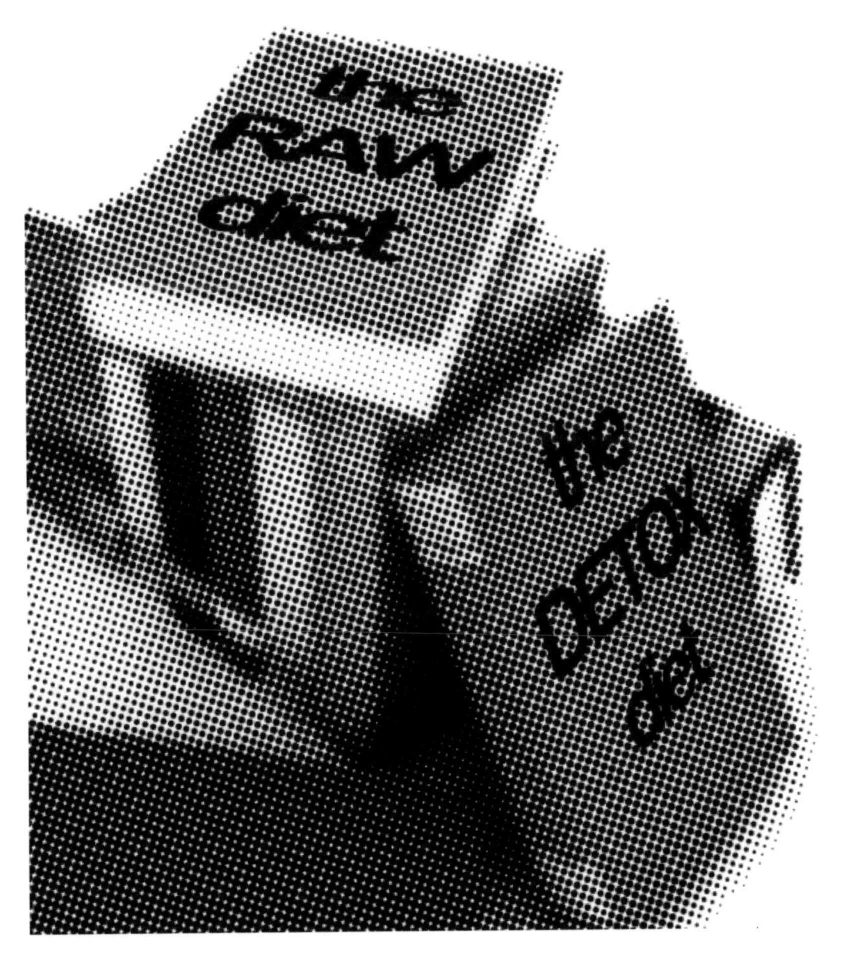

False Promises

Diets that truly disappoint are the diets that guarantee success, offer unrealistic levels of weight or fat loss, focus on only a few *magic* foods or cut calories drastically. The added insult is the requirement to stick rigidly to a programme. A recipe for disaster. Our palates are far too sophisticated to keep shovelling the same foods in for days on end or depriving ourselves of variety and choice. So, how do we spot the diets that are likely to disappoint? The front cover or the *home* page is a good place to start.

Watch out for:-

- Any that are time bound whether it's '2 pounds in 2 minutes' or '2 stones in 2 months' or anything in between.
- Any that promise a flat stomach, slim hips or a great arse.
- Any that guarantee we will drop a dress size or two.
- Any that sing the praises of a single food (banana, grapefruit, chocolate, cabbage, lemon etc.)
- Any that promise we will never be hungry.
- Any that suggest we can eat all we want and still lose weight.

Many *quick fix* diets may deliver in the short term but rarely in the long term but that doesn't mean they are the root of all evil nutritionally speaking.

Some offer gold nuggets of advice that can increase our understanding of what makes good food great for weight loss. Others can kick-start our quest to lose fat if we use what we learn to progress and don't make a beeline for the nearest kebab shop the minute we end the diet. Why so many *quick fix*, *crash* and *boot camp* diets work for so few and sometimes represent a health risk both physically and mentally is discussed in greater depth in the next chapter, *Are You Ready for the Red Carpet?*

Hassle

Other popular diets that come in for regular criticism are the ones that mess around with the balance of food groups. High protein, low carbohydrate, high fibre, low fat, no sugar etc. and most of them are a real hassle. While many are at pains to tell us there's no calorie counting, there is usually some other kind of maths involved. Whether it's points or grams or blueberries or calories, it's still counting and counting equals hassle. The money spinners in this category include the *Atkins*, the *South Beach*, the *Zone*, the *F Plan*, the *Pritikin*, the *Ornish*, the *Fat Smash*, the *Sugar Busters* and *Weight Watchers*.

Then there's *typing*, where we work out our blood type, metabolic type or body type then eat foods that suit and bin those that don't. These are really hard work – more of a mission than a diet, requiring real dedication. And interestingly, all the foods we love are usually on the *bin* list!

Others that fit neatly into the hassle bracket are diets that encourage us to pretend we are not British and adopt the eating practices of countries we may never even have visited. Japan, France, Greece and cities like New York and Los Angeles are favourites. Healthy eating habits of other nations are to be admired and we can learn a lot from them but these diets require a radical change to both our life and our shopping baskets. Radical change is never easy, particularly when it comes to diet.

Lastly, there are the *Raw*, the *Liquid* and the *Detox* diets. These are possibly the biggest hassle of all. Many involve not only counting, dedication and radical change but also time. Time to peel, chop, slice, measure, juice, strain, simmer, chew and sob! Time is precious so unless you have plenty of it and a good helping of iron discipline, these can be an uphill struggle. A better option may be to head off to a retreat somewhere sunny for a week and let someone else do all the peeling, chopping and juicing (recommended retreats and detox camps are at the back of the book).

Investigation into many of the above reveals a number of similarities. They generally propose an *initial phase* where food and drink consumption is greatly reduced. Whether it's calories, carbohydrates, sugar, fat or portions this is the tough part and may reduce many to tears. The *secondary phase* involves a gradual increase in consumption and introduces good wholesome foods, lots of hydrating drinks and of course regular exercise. Then there is the *maintenance phase* which is for life. By this stage we have hopefully learned enough to keep us motivated and success is around the corner. The other common thread is that many diets require a high level of commitment and adherence to the programme and this is where the problem often lies. Sticking to a precise set of rules for a few weeks can be managed, but for life? That's a tall order. The theory is sound but the aforementioned 90% failure rate suggests that it's a whole lot harder in practice.

But there is gold to be found in some of them. The major food groups are usually explained, the importance of vitamin, mineral and fibre rich foods are discussed plus the importance of regular exercise is rarely forgotten. I am not suggesting that this information alone is sufficient to guarantee successful weight loss but what I have discovered is that even when people fail to achieve or maintain desired weight loss they invariably learn something along the way allowing them to be more analytical of fat loss programmes in the future. Knowledge and understanding gives us that power.

To achieve success with any diet, ask yourself the three vital questions and if they don't deliver on all three counts, **don't do it**.

1. What are the potential personal pitfalls and can they be managed/overcome?
2. Do I understand and believe in the principles behind the promised weight/fat loss?
3. Do I have the right attitude to make it work – and last?

So What's Sound?

Slow + Steady

The gospel according to many *experts* is that sustainable weight loss (1-2lbs per week) can only be achieved through sensible calorie reduction. Eat a wide variety of foods from the major food groups supplying essential health-giving nutrients, take regular exercise to build muscle, improve cardiovascular health and burn fat effectively plus drink plenty of water to stay hydrated and facilitate efficient metabolism.

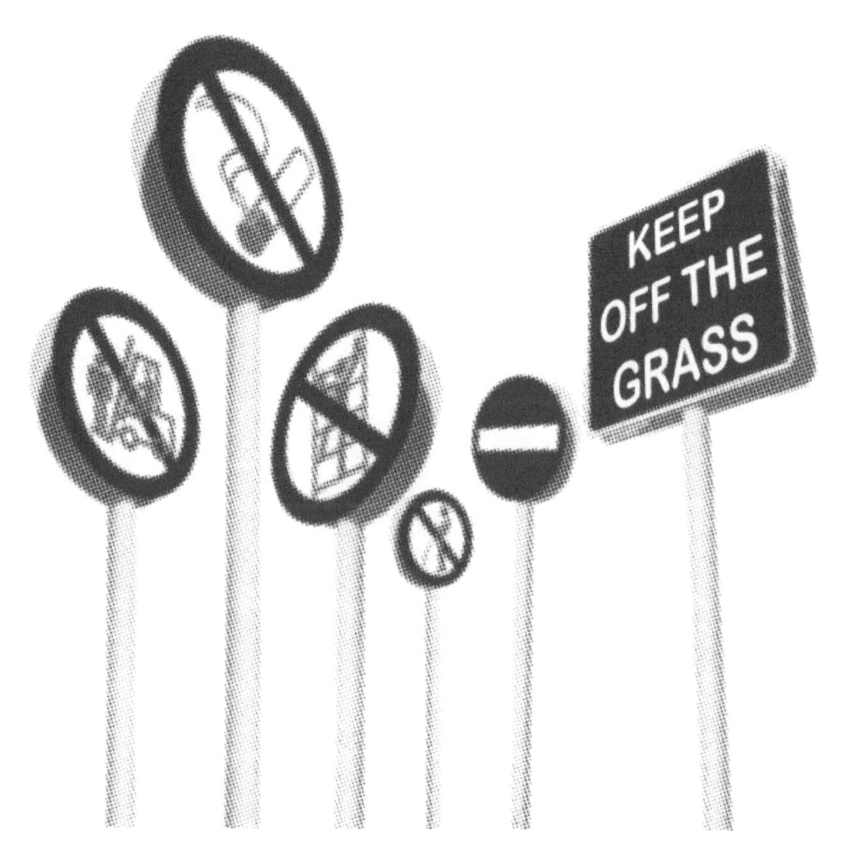

There are as many variations on this *gospel* as there are ways to achieve it but they generally advocate the same principles:-

- Eat more whole foods, eat less refined foods.
- Eat more *good* fats, eat less *bad* fats.
- Eat more *good* carbohydrates, eat less *bad* carbohydrates.
- Eat more beans and lentils, eat less meat.
- Drink more water, drink less coffee and alcohol.
- Avoid junk, processed and fast foods.
- Avoid sweets, biscuits, cakes, fizzy drinks and salty snacks.
- Get back into the kitchen, reduce stress, eat slowly etc.

Good counsel, but is it achievable? Some argue that it is harder to stick to these rules than to stick to some sort of crazy *crash diet* that only allows you lemon, maple syrup and water all day - and there's a lot less shopping!

GI + GL Diets

A relatively new concept which is gaining ground because it really can work. It focuses on blood sugar control. Keeping blood sugar balanced depends not only on what we eat, but also on how and when we eat. Combining low GI/GL carbohydrates with proteins and essential fats and adding exercise helps us feel fuller for longer, tunes up metabolism and burns unwanted fat. If you like a bit of adding, subtracting, multiplying and dividing, it's a winner. Not too hard to stick to once you get your head around it but there are quite a number of rules and if rules don't *float your boat* you could sink!

Natural Foods

Foods free from additives, preservatives, colourings, processing and straight from the ground, tree or bush are believed to boost our natural defences, provide a host of metabolism-boosting enzymes and promote everything from better digestion and elimination to a sharper brain, great skin, hair and nails, healthy bones and even a better sex life. How to fit these diets into a 21st century lifestyle may be the major stumbling block, however.

Healthy Weight Loss

Healthy weight loss is becoming the new *fad* with books and websites cropping up daily. They usually contain phrases like *better life*, *don't diet*, *super health*, *feed your body* etc or are named after the creator, many of whom have been punting the healthy diet angle for years. Plus, most of them have pretty good websites which provide support, forums and recipes galore. Word of warning however; you may find many of them way too prescriptive. But as before, check out the websites and ask yourself the three vital questions before you decide.

So What Rocks?

Curiosity

If you want to be one of the 10% who shed fat for good I recommend you sharpen up your diet detective skills, ignore most of the stuff you have read or heard about *fad* diets and make your own decisions. A *fad* is "a practice or interest followed for a time with exaggerated zeal". It could be a handbag, a book, a movie, a shade of lipstick, a new form of exercise, a fast food craze, a new cocktail, whatever. They are hard to ignore and even harder not to buy into. They swamp the media, are new and exciting and for a period of time they own that enviable position of being the *must have* or the *must do* and we love them.

Where diets differ is that they involve some sort of lifestyle change and that's never as easy as changing your lipstick! But when the latest diet grabs the headlines showing "fantastic results" for some, we all get a little bit hooked. We are desperate and time is short, we need to drop a dress size before our wedding day or we are going on holiday and the thought of baring all is causing us sleepless nights so something has to be done and fast. It has to be worth a try we decide - and after all it's only a few weeks of denial.

But there's always that little nagging doubt. We've launched into these *quick fix* diets before and all we remember is how miserable, tired and hungry we felt. But the weight loss was worth it, even if it didn't last - or was it?

It doesn't have to be that way. A diet can work if it's tailored to our food preferences, our lifestyle, our budget, our energy dips, our cravings and our needs.

So, why should *The Fat Loss Plan* in this book work where others have failed? Because you create your own plan - a diet that works for you. It is designed in such a way that you can tailor it to your lifestyle and preferences. It is easy to understand, easy to believe in and easy to put into practice. And it won't give you attitude, just fat loss. Moreover, it ensures that diet confusion becomes a thing of the past.

Losing body fat can be simple, straightforward and enjoyable when food decisions fit comfortably into our day, not overtake our day. And, NO we are not staring obesity and ill-health in the face unless we ditch those burgers forever, no matter what the *food police* tell us. Food is not only one of life's great pleasures but is also essential to life. We are lucky; we live in a country where food is plentiful and we have the luxury of choice. A diet should never be about depriving ourselves of the foods we love or devoting our lives to sprouts. Life is short and should be fun.

Listening + Learning

Should we stop being curious about diets that hit the bookshelves with new promises or different approaches to weight loss even after we have designed our own sustainable plan? No way! People are inquisitive by nature and the more curious we are, the more we learn about what works or doesn't work for us. Fine-tuning our diet detective skills allows us to uncover a wealth of tips and tricks that can increase our understanding and give us the nutritional edge.

But what about the 10% of dieters who don't fail? Do they all see the light, adopt a healthy lifestyle, learn to say no to *Krispy Kremes* and change their eating habits for life?

Part 1. Chapter Three

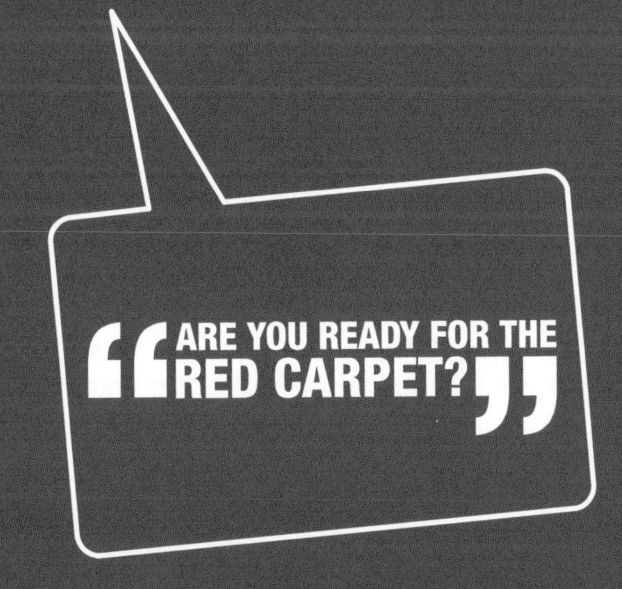

There are over 6 million internet sites dedicated to celebrity diets!

Confused?

Do celebrities actually follow the diets they endorse? One thing is for sure; success now depends not only on their stage and screen skills but also on looking good 24/7. Many celebrities look fabulous and are bursting with health and vitality; others look worryingly skeletal, are possibly undernourished and probably miserable. It's not difficult to imagine how the pressure can get to them when their image is continually being scrutinised - it's tough being a star. So how do they do it and can we learn anything from them?

So What Sucks?

Starvation

Severe calorie restriction is no fun and leaves us starving and the only way we can cope is by having bucket-loads of willpower or by being policed. Celebrities use a variety of tactics to achieve their enviable weight loss or get back into their skinny jeans just weeks after giving birth and many diets have become best sellers through association with the stars (*Maple Syrup, Apple Cider Vinegar, Grapefruit, Cookies, Cabbage Soup, Baby Food, Leech Therapy* (ouch!), *Boiled Eggs* etc.) The temptation to follow them can be strong but consider this. Rapid *weight* loss may be achieved, but *fat* loss is unlikely and side effects are inevitable. Pounding headaches, exhaustion, mood swings, sore joints and a fuzzy brain are sure signs that the body is not happy. However, the feeling of being in control when sticking to any of these regimes can be euphoric and for some, addictive.

One of the most worrying aspects of near starvation or *crash diets* is the promotion of disordered eating patterns. The internet is awash with heart-rending stories and disturbing pictures of people who live with a full-blown eating disorder. Anorexia nervosa and bulimia nervosa are recognised illnesses which can only be treated by professionals and with a great deal of support. They are illnesses that manifest themselves over a period of time as a result of both genetic and environmental factors and there are estimates that up to 4% of young women between the ages of 15 and 24 suffer from one or other or both in their teens and twenties. Furthermore, in one survey of over 4,000 women between the ages of 25 and 45, a staggering 75% reported disordered eating behaviours. That's three out of every four admitting to an unhealthy relationship with either food or their bodies. Unlike anorexia nervosa and bulimia nervosa, disordered eating is not a recognised illness but sure as hell can be regarded as a condition. A condition that can all too quickly arise when we force ourselves to adopt unnatural eating practices which deprive the body of essential nutrients and for some, can lead to eating disorders.

Hard Labour

Another favourite approach with celebrities are *boot camps* where they drop a dress size or two in a week by being physically beaten into submission by a few *hot* marines and living on super-meagre rations - often great food but not much of it. Could this be the route for you? When it works it does so largely due to the fact that all choice is removed. You can learn a lot about yourself in a week when you are tired, hungry and discover muscles you didn't even know you had and every one of them aches from dawn to dusk! Even if you are fit before enrolling at a boot camp, it's a big challenge.

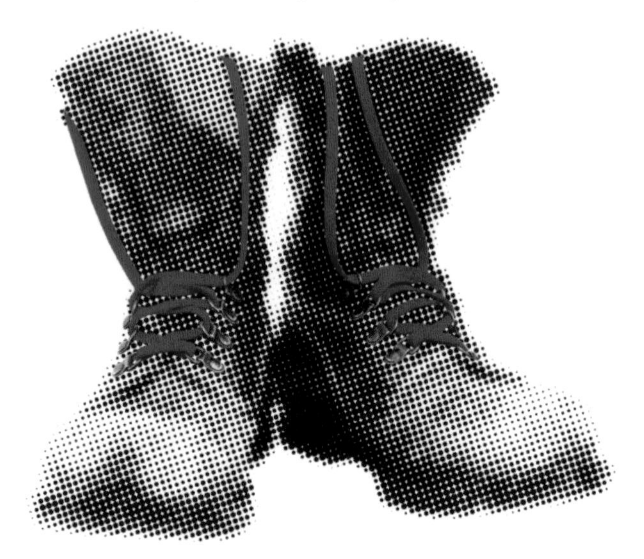

Putting someone else in charge reaps rewards but can it be maintained when stepping back into the real world or is the temptation to pig out on pasta and pastries on our return home too strong? Can eating and exercise habits be overturned in a week? For some it can be a life-changing experience that uncovers a host of reasons why permanent fat loss may have evaded them. The encouragement and advice of the fitness and nutrition teams can prompt *campers* to direct the enthusiasm and drive they display in other aspects of their lives into kicking their weight problem into touch for good. For others, it's just too big a mountain to climb and a month or two down the line they are back to their original dress size and the only thing that has lost weight for good is their credit card. It's worth noting that celebrities rarely pay for this kind of punishment, but you do – and it's not cheap!

So What's Sound?

Possible Health Risks

Crash diets pave the way to yo-yo dieting which may present long-term health risks and depression for some. *Weight cycling* is the scientific term for those who restrict their dietary energy regularly by trying one regime after another in a bid to lose weight. Yo-yo dieters often skip meals, follow seriously low calorie diets to the letter and even stop eating for a time. Initial weight loss is invariably achieved but the body restricts the rate of weight loss after a week or two by slowing down metabolism. Metabolism is the body's food burning system and when calories are limited the body can only cope by going into *preservation mode*. A slower metabolism leads to slower weight loss and muscle tone is often lost. Frustration follows for the yo-yo dieter and more often than not a return to previous eating habits. Weight gain is inevitable because the body responds to the perceived *famine* by ensuring it is prepared to cope with any further deprivation. We are genetically programmed to store energy in order to preserve life. Sadly, this can mean that the yo-yo dieter ends up back on the starting block or worse still heavier than when they started. In the long term *weight cycling* can make future fat loss harder, change where body fat is stored and alter blood pressure. It can also put stress on a number of organs and increase the risk of heart disease. There is also an increased risk of gallstone formation due to a build-up of cholesterol, bile and calcium salts in the gallbladder.

So What Rocks?

It's Fascinating!

There are over 6 million internet sites dedicated to celebrity diets and clicking on just the first few pages reveals a lot. They attract a wealth of conflicting views and criticism but it appears to be an obsession that's here to stay so can we learn something from the less wacky amongst them?

How celebrities achieve red carpet fabulousness is not a new phenomenon. Told that she was too fat for the camera in the mid 1920's, screen goddess Joan Crawford allegedly stuck to a diet of steak, grapefruit and tomatoes for a time and from then on rarely gave in to excess. Vanity Fair magazine reported in February 1936, "She is always conscious of the way that she appears to her public and is continually concerned about her face and figure. When she is working on a picture, she drinks a cup of hot water when she is called at six o'clock, has fruit juice and coffee for breakfast, a salad for lunch and dinner without white bread or potatoes. She drinks wine now and then, but no hard liquor". Joan Crawford knew what was required to be a star and the magazines of the day couldn't get enough of her. She didn't endorse a *diet* programme and she didn't spend copious hours in the gym. But then there were few if any gurus to the stars then – would she hire one now?

So, what has changed? The big difference is in the word diet. Joan Crawford probably regarded her food choices as a diet in the true meaning of the word; a way of life. A way of life that included foods that gave her energy, helped her focus, fed her beautiful complexion and kept her at the top of her game. Diet no longer means a way of life. Diet no longer means occasionally cutting back when our waistbands feel a little tight after Christmas or watching what we eat for a few weeks before going on holiday. It now means embarking on regimes that restrict the energy we get from food with the sole intention of losing a substantial amount of body weight. It means altering our normal pattern of eating and more often than not, feeling deprived and hungry and dreaming of *Krispy Kremes*! And once the desired weight loss is achieved, a joyous return to the foods we love and because the body has been in what it perceives as *famine mode*, weight gain, prompting the search for another diet or accepting defeat.

The constant barrage of photographs in the media of super-skinny celebrities who reportedly live on thin air, coffee and cigarettes, maple syrup, edamame beans or acai berries and use all manner of diet pills, laxatives and appetite suppressants are a stark reminder of just how detrimental continued calorie restriction can be to health.

So why do some of the regimes work for celebrities but not for the rest of us? There are four major reasons:-

1. They have a huge incentive to lose weight. They are paid fat sums of money to look good on screen, stage or catwalk.
2. They get plenty of support. They rarely make the mistake of going it alone. They hire personal trainers, healthy eating gurus, life coaches, hypnotists and a host of other *experts* to keep them on target.
3. They get paid handsomely to endorse weight loss programmes (TV and radio appearances, website profiles, newspaper and magazine articles, product and supplement endorsement etc.) whether they adopt them or not.
4. They often have meals delivered. These meals are healthy, portioned, balanced and beautifully presented and seriously limit the temptation to reach for the biscuit tin or scoff the children's leftovers. This can be an expensive route to weight loss but most of them can afford it*.

These points are crucial if we are tempted to buy into the celebrities' alleged routines. If they do indeed follow wacky, near-starvation diets it's likely that it is for a particular event (a new movie, TV series, photo shoot etc.) with a clear time limit. As weight loss has to be maintained and a healthy and toned look is as important to their careers as being slim they move on to a more manageable, long-term programme.

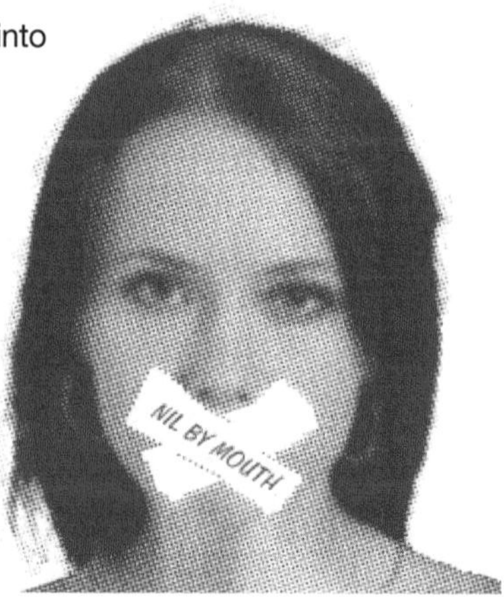

Secrets of Success

We can learn a lot from the stars that adopt the less dramatic of these diets. There are certain recommendations common to many that are a must in any *Fat Loss Plan*, most of which are discussed in greater depth in later chapters.

- They drink plenty of water. Water is essential for every chemical reaction that takes place in the body. Dehydration slows reactions down and can result in a 20% drop in energy levels - the body needs energy to burn fat. Water is also a great hunger buster which is an added bonus.
- They don't forget breakfast. Refuelling first thing in the morning kick-starts our metabolism, provides energy, keeps hunger at bay and reduces cravings for sugary, salty and fatty snacks.
- They eat little and often. When it comes to eating to burn fat it is important to avoid energy dips during the day – this is a real danger zone.
- They bin the salt cellar. The modern diet contains too much sodium and too little potassium causing fluid retention and increasing the risk of high blood pressure. Too much salt can also lead to dramatic and frustrating weight fluctuations.
- They eat fat to lose fat. This is one of the great fat busting tactics that serial dieters rarely take on board. Such is the bad press fats have received over the past thirty years that many dieters adopt the 'avoid all fats' principle. Wrong. Essential fats, Omega 3s in particular are vital for the brain, energy production, our skin, our sex hormones and long term fat loss and should become our dietary best friends.
- They eat raw foods (fruits, vegetables, sprouts, nuts, seeds etc.) Delicious, colourful and packed with nutrients they increase our water intake, promote good digestion, are bursting with protective antioxidants and keep the dreaded munchies at bay.
- They control their portions. Eating until we are only 80% full results in us consuming less calories per day – 700kcals less per day means 21,000kcals less per month, 252,000kcals per year and over a million in 5 years!
- They exercise every day. The importance of daily exercise cannot be overstated when it comes to improving health and fitness but can be difficult to fit into a busy life. There are lots of ways to get more physical on a daily basis and thankfully it's not all about pounding the treadmill for hours on end. See chapter 15, *Your Body is Made of Moving Parts, So Move Them.*

* if you can afford it for a few weeks/months, having meals prepared and delivered to your door can be a great way to kick start fat loss. They have been popular in the US for a number of years and are beginning to be taken-up in the UK. Some are great, others are not. The best offer balanced, portioned, nutritious and exciting meals and snacks that not only take shopping and preparation time out of your life but also provide opportunities to experiment with food combinations that can form the basis of a long term eating plan. Some also have support teams to keep you focused and answer your dietary queries. See the back of the book for contact details.

Part 1. Chapter Four

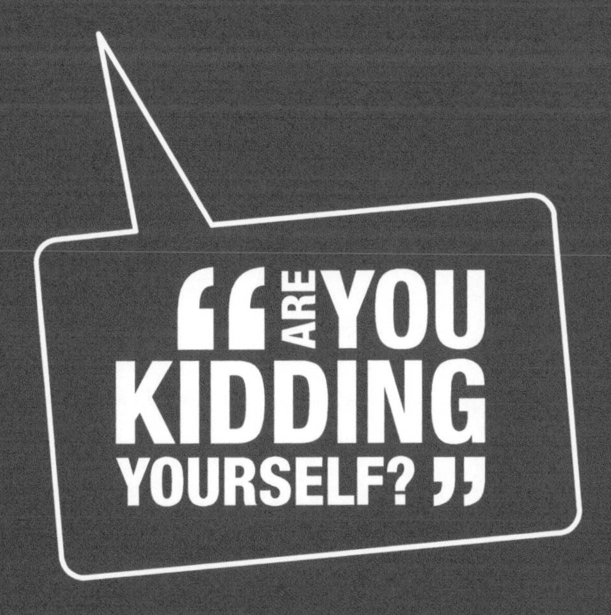

If it is banned, promises a lot, offered for free or guarantees weight loss don't touch it!

Confused?

The diet pill is still king when it comes to dieting. They account for well over half the weight loss searches on the internet and are a huge money-spinner. Do any of them work, are they effective or dangerous or just another pipe dream which promises a lot, delivers little and leaves us hopeless, helpless and looking for another solution?

The estimated spend on diet pills in the US was 43.6 billion dollars in 2008 and although figures for the UK are less well-recorded, £12 million was quoted in 2006. There are a staggering 7 million plus sites offering news, research, case studies and advice but regretfully the majority are devoted to encouraging rather than deterring people from signing up.

You can buy over the counter diet pills by the dozen in sports emporiums, supermarkets and health shops; you can also get a wide selection from therapists and private practitioners. Appetite suppressants and fat burners are favourites and predominate. You can also get a prescription from your GP for the weight loss drug, orlistat (*Xenical*) which is the only weight loss medication approved by the NHS or a course of *Alli* (a form of orlistat) which is the first and only non-prescription weight loss aid to be licensed for use throughout Europe from your local chemist. But you must have a body mass index (BMI) of 28 plus or a medical condition which presents particular health risks to qualify. So, if you don't meet the criteria, are there other options?

Diet pills divide into three groups:-

- **Pills licensed as medicines in the UK** – these are approved by the Government and rigorously tested for safety and effectiveness.
- **Herbal remedies/food supplements** – these are not licensed as medicines but as foods and are therefore less rigorously tested which allows some manufacturers to make weight loss claims which are sometimes based on limited research. They are however subject to British/European laws on safety and efficacy and include ingredients which may increase metabolic rate, control appetite, reduce fat absorption or act as diuretics or laxatives.
- **Slimming pills available on the internet** – some are legitimate, some are loosely regulated and some are illegal and potentially dangerous.

Despite being banned in Britain there are products freely available online that should more accurately be described as *diet drugs.* A legal loophole allows overseas chemists to peddle them without conscience and it is estimated that there are over 2,000 websites selling drugs without prescription to customers worldwide in an industry worth £30 billion. They are often very powerful with lengthy lists of unpleasant side effects and often frightening health consequences when used long term.

So What Sucks?

The dangers far outweigh any benefits

Amphetamine-type diet pills are not new. They've been around in various guises since the 1960's and the reason they were taken off the market in the UK, the US and many European countries is because they are highly addictive and can cause not only multiple side effects but also extreme changes in behaviour. People took them innocently before they were banned and sadly still do thinking they are an easy way to lose weight. They work by stimulating the central nervous system, mimicking the natural effect of adrenalin by increasing the heart rate and suppressing the appetite. Euphoria and increased energy levels are often listed as additional benefits by the unscrupulous sellers but insomnia, hallucinations, mood swings, anxiety, paranoia and violent behaviour are common side effects and because of the extreme stress on the heart and raised blood pressure, convulsions, heart attacks, strokes and even death can result. Tragically, the unsuspecting are still wooed by the weight loss promise.

Banned amphetamine-type pills are not the only ones to watch out for. There are also drugs being touted for their ability to prevent the absorption of fat. Under prescription and alongside a balanced diet and exercise programme some fat absorbers have shown reasonable weight loss results. But without guidance many can cause nutrient deficiencies which may result in fatigue at best, bouts of depression, confusion and menstrual mayhem at worst and seriously messy and embarrassing episodes of sudden and uncontrolled diarrhoea – not a pretty scene.

The word *anorectic* is sometimes used to describe pills that may promote weight loss. Don't be fooled, they are drugs. Before any drug is accepted for general use by the Department of Health and prescribed by health professionals it must go through rigorous, repetitive and costly testing, so rest assured that if it is later taken off the market it is for very good reason. Only a professional who has the appropriate training, knowledge and experience can evaluate our health status and decide on our suitability. Self medication or *'cocktailing'*, where additional drugs are taken to alleviate the side effects from pills already being used leads to metabolic imbalances which are unlikely to result in the weight loss craved, health conditions that can have serious long term consequences and the sort of frustration and negativity that prevents dieters from relishing the advantages they imagine a slimmer body may reap.

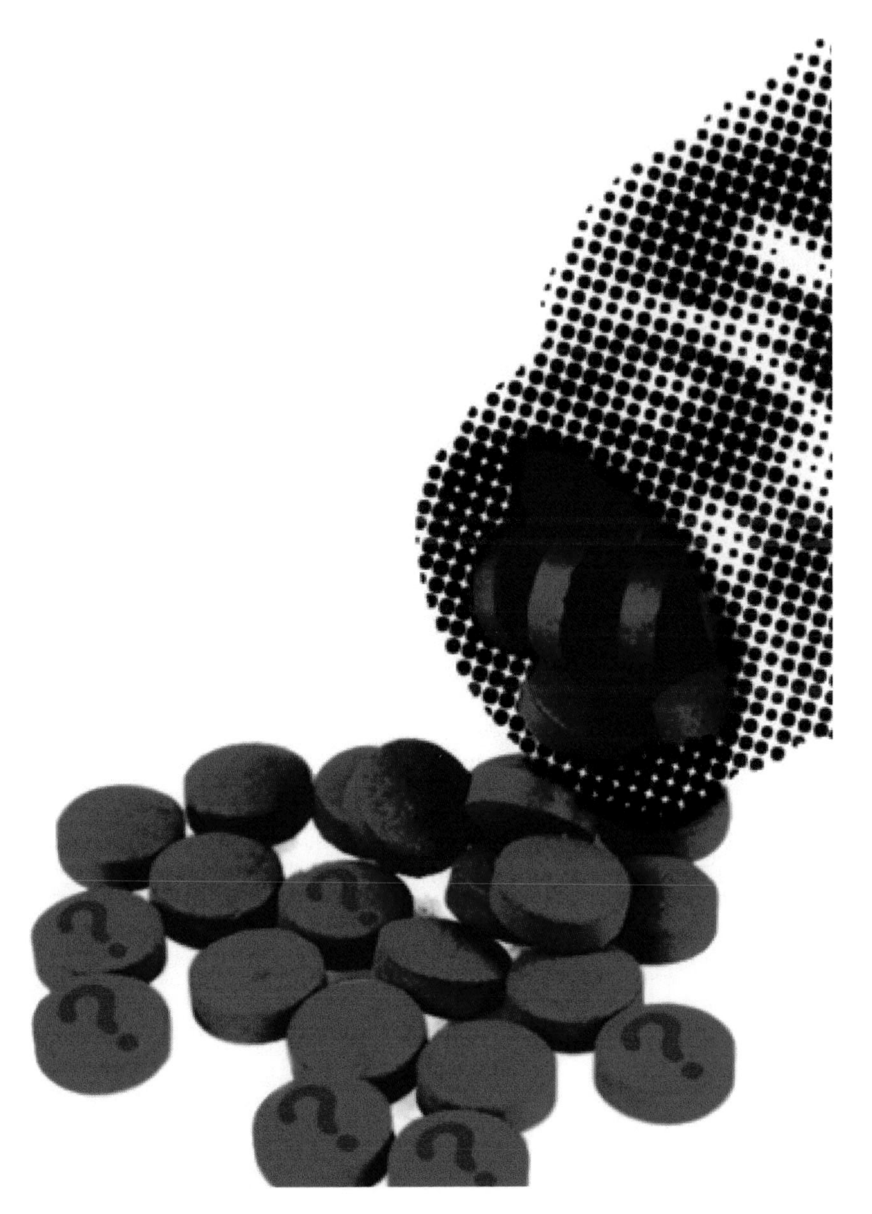

If it is a banned substance, don't touch it. If it promises a lot don't touch it. If it is offered for free, don't touch it. If it guarantees weight loss without changing eating habits or exercising, don't touch it.

If any of them worked long term and had no alarming side effects or threats to health they would have made it into the A-list and stayed there. If you are tempted to buy into the hype peddled on the internet by unscrupulous pharmacies do yourself a huge favour and do some research before even considering hitting the *buy* button. There are fewer sites dedicated to empowering us than sites dedicated to ruining our health and stealing our money but they are there – seek them out. Diet pills are a huge issue, they reek of danger and the subject definitely merits a lot more than a chapter but forewarned is forearmed.

Addiction + Overdose

Anyone who decides that any of the above might work, parts with their hard-earned cash and takes the recommended dose may lose weight in the short term. Then what happens? With luck, they decide they can't cope with the side effects and sling them down the toilet – a good decision. Alternatively, they ignore the tremors, mood swings, digestive upset etc. and press on because they are relishing the weekly weight loss - the promise is delivering and after years of restrictive diets, punishing exercise routines and the rest, the fat is falling off. Then hooked, they order another batch then another. Addiction to diet pills is easy, understandable and rife. Why? Chiefly, because fear of weight gain and the possibility of unpleasant withdrawal symptoms drives many people to continue usage despite potential health risks. Regular users often make few changes to their diet, believing that these concoctions can trick the body into continually suppressing appetite, speeding up metabolism or absorbing fat more effectively. But the body is far too sophisticated to be repeatedly fooled and as with severe calorie restriction, biochemical coping mechanisms leap into action.

Substance abuse of any kind creates extra work for the liver as toxic by-products must be neutralised before being eliminated from the body but the liver is not invincible; a lack of essential nutrients and too many toxins to cope with impair its performance. The liver's role in fat burning is significant and its health impacts on its efficiency. In short, diet pill addiction poses not only a serious threat to health but may ultimately cause weight gain. They are NOT the answer.

The other great temptation is to take more than the recommended dose. If two a day produce the sort of weight loss the dieter yearns for, perhaps three or four might work better or more quickly. Taking diet pills regularly is counter-productive; overdosing on them is dangerous. What may start as unpleasant or irritating side effects when following the instructions to the letter can all too quickly result in hospitalisation. Stomach pumping, cardiac arrests and bowel dysfunction are not uncommon and simply not worth it.

What about over the counter 'slimming' pills?

Yes, many of them are natural but how natural is it to take huge doses of a concentrated substance that grows in the ground, on a bush or as part of the bark or root of a tree three to four times a day? Regular coffee drinkers are familiar with the jitters that occur when a few cups are downed during the morning without having had breakfast. Many over the counter slimming pills work in the same way. Like caffeine, many are stimulants and whilst they can suppress appetite, superficially increase energy levels, lift mood and produce the sort of high that may keep us going for hours they also bring on the energy crash that prompts the need for another hit to *stay in the zone*.

Some find that living on nothing but coffee, cigarettes and alcohol for days on end keeps hunger at bay effectively. Eureka they think, they are not hungry, they don't eat, they lose weight and it's all good. They know instinctively that it's probably not very good for their health but they reason they'll get that all sorted out once they have lost a few pounds. Does the body agree? Absolutely not. It's starving – starving for nutrients to feed the brain, the immune system, bones and organs and make no mistake; the body will find nutrients from wherever it can because survival is its number one priority. The muscles are called upon to give up stored energy resulting in the skeletal look which makes no sense but sadly many crave. This kind of energy restriction carries with it a whole host of threats and the strong possibility of future ill-health that may be irreversible.

Taking diet pills regularly is counter-productive; overdosing on them is dangerous.

Caffeine, guarana, white willow bark, synephrine, ginseng, ephedrine, GABA and a host of other natural and herbal extracts are all stimulants and while innocuous and sometimes health-giving in modest doses and under supervision, can cause headaches, nausea, insomnia, restlessness, excitation, tremors, irregular heartbeats, dizziness, fainting and stomach ulcers if taken regularly throughout the day, particularly when quick weight loss is the goal. Countless studies show that because they are natural and therefore deemed to be harmless, addiction and overdosing rarely cross the dieter's mind. To make matters worse, laxatives and diuretics are often added to the mix to hasten weight loss. The sales pitch is often that overweight people may be loaded with toxins which need clearing and retaining water which could be foiling their efforts. Don't fall into this trap. There are some excellent herbal and nutritional products on the market which may prompt the body to metabolise foods more efficiently, help to remove toxins from fat stores and reduce water retention but as before, self diagnosis and self medication is discouraged as this route can result in a lot of spend, little result and worrying health consequences. There are professionals who can tailor a programme to fit weight loss aims and make them work – seek them out (recommendations at the back of the book).

Diet Patches

Permanent weight loss can't be achieved with a patch. It's a neat idea though. Trans-dermal patches have had some success with hormone replacement and nicotine addiction but the notion that herbal or nutritionally-active ingredients can be absorbed through the skin and encourage the body to burn fat, decrease appetite, eliminate toxins, reduce water retention or fatigue is still just that - a notion. Watch this space however; it could be a reality in years to come. For now, don't waste your money.

What else is out there?

Slimming wraps, plastic pants, body toning and fitness pads, slimming creams, caffeine tights etc. On the back of a good eating and exercise programme some may tone up the skin and/or encourage fluid loss which may boost the feel good factor before a night on the town but they all come with a price tag. A new pair of shoes may achieve the same effect!

So What's Sound?

Consult Your Doctor

Most GPs are extremely concerned about the increasing number of overweight and clinically obese patients in their practice. They know the associated health risks, they recognise that excess weight puts a strain on the heart and joints and they are there to help.

There is currently one drug available in the UK that is specifically designed and licensed for medication as a weight loss aid but only on prescription. Orlistat *(Xenical)* works by reducing the amount of fat the body absorbs from food. Clinical trials have shown this drug to be effective in tandem with a healthy diet and exercise programme. The same applies to *Alli* (a reduced dose of orlistat) which is the only non-prescription weight loss aid licensed for use in the UK and available from pharmacies.

Successful fat loss has been achieved by many on orlistat so if you have been battling with your weight for years and are willing to adhere to the prescribed programme, make an appointment with your doctor or pharmacist today. The added bonus is that before *Xenical* is prescribed by your doctor he/she will endeavour to uncover any health or lifestyle issues that may be thwarting your fat loss goal. Similarly, your local pharmacist will determine your health status using a questionnaire and measure your BMI before you can purchase a course of *Alli*. If he/she has any concerns you will be referred to your doctor. If you qualify for either of these medications you will be given a diet and exercise programme to follow, guidance on use and lots of support.

It can be awkward and embarrassing to go to your doctor with a weight problem but if you believe they really want to help it can change your life. Alternatively, if you suspect they don't understand the physical and emotional issues you are dealing with by being overweight, change your doctor.

Consult a Nutritional Therapist

The reasons why people can't lose weight or maintain an initial weight loss are many and varied. Health conditions, digestive issues, intolerance to certain foods, a sluggish liver, metabolic interference from regular medication, hormone imbalances or a depressed immune system are just a few that may have an impact. A nutritional therapist will discuss symptoms, health history, lifestyle and eating habits then design a personal programme to suit. The expression 'one man's meat is another man's poison' is overused but never truer than when it comes to food. Sadly, nutritional therapy is not available through the NHS and many people simply can't afford private treatment. Others regard it as an indulgence but when you consider that the UK spend on over the counter medications for colds, flu, menstrual problems, weight loss etc. is around £3bn per annum (that's £60 per person), one consultation with a therapist may save money in the long term. Criticism has been levelled at nutritional therapists and some regard them merely as *supplement pushers*. Unfair on many counts. The goal of most of these professionals is to correct health imbalances before they have an opportunity to manifest themselves as diagnosable diseases and there is certainly no lack of evidence that they improve the health and wellbeing of many.

Your health is your choice. Should you decide to go down this route, do your homework and find a recognised and properly trained therapist.

There are recommendations at the back of the book.

So What Rocks?

Calcium

A diet deficient in calcium increases our risk of brittle bones in later life and whilst it is in no way the only player, extensive research over many years has shown that it plays a vital role in skeletal health. Over the last ten years however, the role calcium plays in fat metabolism has merited a great deal of interest. It appears that this *bone-strengthener* may also be a *fat-buster*. This has led many researchers not only to review existing data but also to conduct further research in an effort to uncover the important role calcium might play in achieving and maintaining a healthy weight. There is no conclusive evidence as yet but there are suggestions that it could be significant.

Analysis of studies to date offer some interesting theories as to why:-

Calcium may inhibit the action of an enzyme, *fatty acid synthase* which encourages fat storage in the body. Diets that are low in calcium (less than 600mg per day) have been found to result in over twice the amount of fat being stored to those providing medium (600mg – 1000mg) or high levels (1000mg plus).

It has also been suggested that increased calcium in the diet may reduce the transport of fat from the intestine to the bloodstream. When calcium binds with bile acids an increase in faecal fat excretion has been noted and less fat in the bloodstream means less fat is stored. However, fats are an important energy source, they insulate our organs and help the body absorb and transport the vitamins A, D, E and K through the bloodstream. It has yet to be ascertained whether this process allows the body to determine between the fats we need and aid their absorption and those that lead to weight gain and ill-health. Further research will hopefully provide greater understanding.

There is also some evidence that when calcium levels in the body are low the brain detects this and stimulates feelings of hunger. These hunger pangs cause us to eat more in an attempt to increase calcium levels. Conversely, good to optimum levels send signals to the brain communicating that we are full, suppressing the desire to eat more.

The current recommended daily calcium intake is set with skeletal health as the endpoint but studies of bone remains of our earliest ancestors indicate that around twice this amount of calcium was ingested from nuts, seeds, plants, meat and fish. To build and maintain strong bones we need not only calcium but also magnesium, vitamin D, boron, manganese, molybdenum, vitamin K, zinc, copper, vitamin B6 and the Omega 3 and Omega 6 fatty acids. The Palaeolithic diet of our early ancestors comprised of red meat and birds (and they ate every part of the animal including the organs), fish and shellfish (bones, heads, the lot), root vegetables, sea vegetables, green leafy plants and bird eggs (including the shells). This provided them with good levels of all of the above vitamins and minerals. And of course their active lifestyle further enhanced bone growth.

Many studies suggesting a possible link between calcium levels and weight loss concentrate on either dairy products or calcium supplementation (both industries are sure to gain financial reward should the proof be conclusive) but from a nutritional point of view this may be a red herring. Milk is a valuable source of calcium up until about the age of 18 when we are still growing but thereafter it can have a negative effect on the body. The protein in milk can acidify the blood and our bodies are forced to extract calcium from our bones to counteract the acidity. Furthermore milk fat can contribute to inflammation within the body and the promotion of an intolerance to milk sugars for some which reduces the likelihood of fat loss.

Also, there is a danger that in a bid to hasten fat burning some people decide that a daily calcium supplement is all that is required but too much of any substance in the body is as detrimental to long term health as is too little so until further studies are completed and the calcium/weight loss connection is proven, natural bio-yoghurt, small fish with bones (whitebait, anchovies, sardines), tinned sardines and salmon, prawns and shrimps, beans, seeds, green leafy vegetables, dried fruits and tofu are the best sources and should feature regularly in our diet. There are suggestions on how to include these foods in your diet on a daily basis in chapter 14, *Lots of 'Eats'*.

Some people have difficulty including some or all of these foods in their diet because they simply don't like them and may wish to consider a supplement but calcium supplementation on its own is not recommended. A supplement should always include magnesium and vitamin D which are vital for the regulation and metabolism of calcium in the body (recommended suppliers are at the back of the book).

Omega 3 Fatty Acids

These feed the fat burning furnace and may aid fat loss in three ways:-

- They form the building blocks of certain hormone-like chemicals which help the kidneys get rid of excess water - fat is often retained in water.
- They increase metabolic rate and consequently energy production which is exactly the opposite of what happens when we cut calories or fat from our diet drastically.
- Because of increased energy levels, people are more likely to be active and build muscle which further increases metabolic rate, helping to make fat loss permanent.

Research into the amazing properties of both Omega 3s and Omega 6s has provided a wealth of knowledge over the past twenty years and is ongoing **BUT WE CAN'T MAKE THESE FATTY ACIDS IN THE BODY, WE HAVE TO GET THEM FROM FOOD.** Omega 3s in particular are one of the big secrets to permanent fat loss.

Flax seeds offer the best levels of Omega 3s and can easily be incorporated into our diet. Other seeds, some nuts and oily fish are also good sources. There's a lot more information on their fat busting qualities and where to find them in chapter 6, *A Little Knowledge is Not a Dangerous Thing* and ways to include them on a daily basis are in chapter 14, *Lots of 'Eats'*. As before, some people struggle to get these foods into their diet in the early stages and may wish to consider a supplement.

There are also a number of nutritional supplements that have been found, in conjunction with lifestyle changes to encourage weight loss.

These Include:-

- **Conjugated Linoleic Acid** (CLA) – a growing body of research in the US and Europe shows that CLA reduces body fat and increases lean tissue.
- **Chromium** – preliminary research in animals and humans suggests that chromium picolinate increases fat loss by helping to maintain healthy blood sugar levels and curb cravings.
- **Hydroxycitric Acid** (HCA) – animal research indicates that HCA can suppress appetite and induce weight loss when taken before meals.
- **L-Carnitine** – preliminary studies suggest l-carnitine may be beneficial for fat loss when taken on a long term basis in combination with regular exercise.
- **Spirulina** – thought to nourish the thyroid gland which can be under-active in some overweight people.
- **5-HTP** – may play a role in raising *serotonin* levels which in turn reduces appetite.
- **7-Keto** – the association with weight loss is believed to be due to 7-Keto's ability to raise levels of T3, a thyroid hormone that plays a major role in metabolic rate.
- **Pyruvate** – has been noted to raise metabolic rate during the metabolism of protein and carbohydrate.
- **Fibre** – some studies show that supplementation with a source of fibre reduces appetite which in turn may influence satiety (the feeling of fullness) and weight loss.

Whilst the above have shown encouraging results in a number of studies, research is still in its infancy. In an effort to determine whether there may be one that can help burn fat more efficiently, the overriding recommendation is to consult a health professional. There are so many reasons why supplementation of any kind of *weight loss accelerator* may or may not work and self medication is not the way to go. It's all too easy to confuse our metabolism and not only will weight loss not result, but we could find ourselves a great deal lighter of pocket.

Part 1. Chapter Five

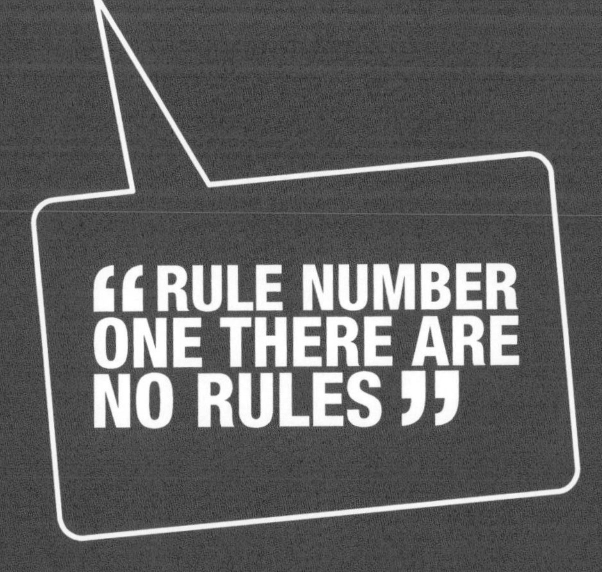

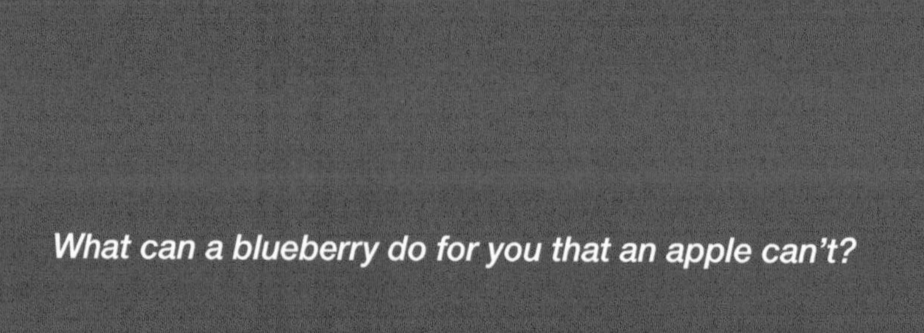
What can a blueberry do for you that an apple can't?

Confused?

Huge tomes have been written on why dieting makes us fat and why diets don't work but it appears many of us just ain't listening! Perhaps we are listening but don't like the message and are still on a quest for the illusive diet that's going to ensure weight loss for good while still enjoying the foods we love. Could it happen? Nutritional science is galloping along at a pace with the antioxidant, fat burning, energy-boosting, immunity-enhancing powers of certain foodstuffs being researched and reported daily. Chocolate and red wine have already leapt up the charts, so what's to say some of our favourites may not be next? Whether to include every food that has been proven to have special powers into your life and how to do it can all too quickly become yet another stress. They demand pages of media coverage and yards of supermarket shelving. Will ignoring them seriously compromise long-term health and undermine the chance of losing fat for good?

So What Sucks?

Blueberries!

They certainly pack a punch nutritionally but are they *super*? If you like them and can afford to sling them regularly on your morning cereal, go ahead but not just because of their perceived *super-powers* or the claims that they may boost weight loss. The same goes for spinach and walnuts and pomegranates and an increasing list of *super* foods. According to one market analyst, sales of blueberries rocketed by £55 million in just two years – an amazing 132% increase, as consumers became aware of the positive publicity surrounding their health benefits. That's a lot of blueberries to force down! What makes little sense from a fat loss perspective is that we often get carried along on the crest of the *super* foods wave without questioning the science behind it. What can a blueberry do for us that an apple can't?

Do these *super* nutrients that are bursting from every berry somehow make for a more filling, fat-busting snack than a banana?

Progress is everything. When scientists tell us that certain foods may extend our lives, shore up our defences or help us shed fat who are we to argue? Some *super* foods have earned extensive research and appear to be rich in nutrients that may boost the health of body cells keeping them fighting fit, others contain substances that may prompt more efficient metabolism but a *super* fit, *super* healthy body demands a great deal more than a shopping basket filled with *super* foods. Research can only be undertaken with adequate funding and in many cases this is supplied by corporations and associations that have a vested interest in uncovering the *super* nutrients in their products which allows them to market them as health-enhancing foods. A somewhat cynical view perhaps but worth consideration when we are faced with so much choice and so many conflicting views.

Fresh produce on sale at our local Farmers' Market is unlikely to have benefited from funding to rubber-stamp its nutritional superiority but the freshness, care and attention taken in getting it from soil to sale and the taste is enough to convince most of us that certification simply isn't required. *Super* food is fresh food that provides the full spectrum of nutrients required to keep us strong and healthy and the list should never be reduced to ten, twenty or even fifty.

What earns many foods their *super* food label is the wealth of antioxidants they provide. Antioxidants are micronutrients that are found in almost every food we eat but many are destroyed by cooking which makes raw and lightly-cooked plant foods our richest source. Plants have developed protection from the environment and disease, a kind of *security blanket* which keeps their defences strong and when we eat them we ingest these micronutrients and benefit from their protective properties. One of our biggest health threats is the now well-documented damage that can be caused by *free radicals*. Few had even heard the term until recently but we are now regularly reminded that they should be regarded as the enemy. But what are they and why do they pose such a threat?

Oxygen is essential to life but can also be the devil in disguise by its very nature. Just as a match won't burn without oxygen neither can we burn the food we eat to release its energy without oxygen. All atoms ideally have an even number of electrons in their outer orbit for stability but when the inner food-burning fire is raging and oxygen is playing its vital role, sparks fly and atoms can lose their electrons. A *free radical* is an atom that has lost an electron and has become unstable and unpredictable. They are *free* because they are at liberty to roam, looking for a new electron to make them stable again and they are *radical* because they will steal an electron from another atom at random. This creates a damaging domino effect because every time an atom is robbed of an electron it becomes *free* and is forced to go on the hunt. Thousands of *free radical* reactions can

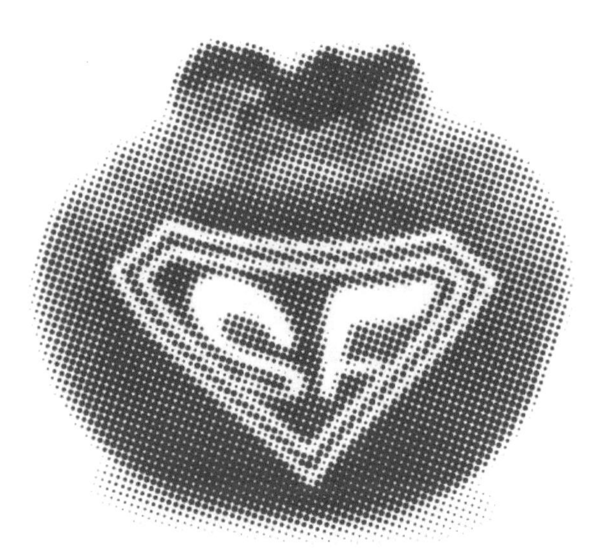

occur in seconds threatening not only the integrity of the outer membranes of our body cells but also their DNA which can alter cell behaviour, reduce effectiveness and compromise our health. *Free radicals* are involved in many diseases including coronary artery disease, Alzheimer's, arthritis, cataracts and some cancers.

Antioxidants are the *protective parents* that form a shield around the cells. This shield absorbs *free radicals* which are neutralised, lose their destructive energy and are safely excreted in urine. If you cut an apple in half and leave one half uncovered for 20 minutes you can see the *free radical* damage occurring. The apple starts to go brown and dries up because it reacts with the oxygen in the air causing *free radicals* to be formed. If you soak the other half in lemon juice however, it retains its creamy, white colour and texture. This is because it has been protected by the vitamin C in lemon juice. Vitamin C is a powerful antioxidant.

The more antioxidant-rich foods we introduce into our diet the better our defence. Fruits and vegetables are the major players but nuts and whole grains do a fairly impressive job too. But, just as one talented striker can't win the game on his own, one antioxidant-rich *super* food can't do the job alone. The rest of the team are vital, so if we want to ensure that our antioxidant shield is strong we have to get the whole team of fruits, vegetables, nuts and whole grains into our diet. And don't forget the humble banana!

So What's Sound?

Change Your Habits

Don't think diet, think change. When we change our approach to weight control, change the way we think about food, say no and mean it, stick with a plan and don't give in to temptation, fat loss and improved health are likely to follow. Living a life full of health-giving foods, getting eight hours sleep every night, exercising regularly in the fresh air and managing stress become part of our daily routine. All we have to do is bin the cigarettes, coffee, boozy nights out with friends, snacks, treats, fast food and late night takeaways.

Making major changes results in improved health and permanent fat loss for many. If we believe we can do it, we can and once on this road we may never stray because when we rediscover the kind of energy we haven't had since childhood and manage to fight off 'bugs' and viruses that threaten us, we don't want to go back. Embracing change and learning as much as we can gives us that power. There are a great many books dedicated to helping people achieve optimum health and many make fascinating and inspirational reading (there are a few mentioned at the back of the book).

This book however, is more geared to those of us who struggle with the word no, find radical change difficult and want to shout from the rooftops that life

without a few of our favourites just isn't living! But, with a few strategic changes, fat loss goals can be achieved – read on!

So What Rocks?

The Futility of Repetition

Repetition works for exercise and learning French verbs but not for long term fat loss. Many diets and weight loss programmes are criticised because there is a limited choice of meals and snacks so they quickly become boring. Others fail to succeed because there is too much choice and they become confusing and complicated. We are creatures of habit so in a bid to lose fat it is important to determine just how much freedom of choice we want and how much routine we need. In an effort to help you decide, there are some characteristics you may identify with in chapter 9, *Are You a Rule Maker, a Rule Breaker or a Disciple?*

Try this

Here are three lists of foods that get top marks for their nutritional goodness. One for carbohydrates, one for proteins and one for fats. Select one or two from each list for each meal and snack to create a day's eating plan (aim for a breakfast, a mid morning snack, a lunch, a mid afternoon snack and an evening meal).

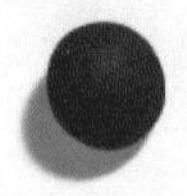

Carbohydrates

Oats, Porridge, Oatcakes, Brown bread, Whole wheat pasta, Brown basmati rice, Muesli, Whole grain cereals, Cereal Bars, Rye Bread, Rye Crackers, Ryvita, Pumpernickel, Tacos, Nachos, Corn Chips, Popcorn, Pita Pockets, Tortillas, Couscous, Bulghur wheat, Sweet Potatoes, Beans (baked, kidney, butter, black eyed, flageolet, haricot etc), Lentils (red, green, yellow), Legumes (chickpeas, broad beans, runner beans, peas), Pumpkin, Squash (butternut, acorn etc), Fruits, Vegetables.

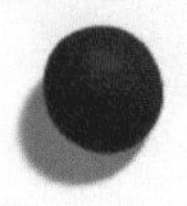

Protein

Fish, Shellfish, Lean Meats, Skinless Poultry, Game, Eggs, Cheese, Beans, Lentils and Legumes (see carbohydrates), Low-fat milk, Yoghurt, Crème Fraiche, Dairy Alternatives (rice milk, oat milk, almond milk etc.), Tofu, Soya milk, Soya spread and yoghurt, Nuts, Seeds.

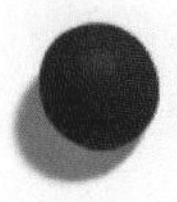

Fats

Oily fish (sardines, mackerel, salmon, trout, herring, kippers, anchovies, fresh tuna, eel, whitebait, swordfish), Nuts (almonds, walnuts, hazelnuts, Brazils, cashew nuts, macadamia nuts, pistachios, pine nuts), Seeds (flax, linseed, sesame, pumpkin, sunflower, safflower, hemp), Olive Oil, Nut and Seed oils and butters, Coconut Milk and cream, Omega 3-rich eggs, Natural live yoghurt, Skimmed and semi-skimmed milk, Crème fraiche (low fat).

Here are a couple of suggestions:-

Mid Morning Snack - Oatcakes, hummus and a bag of mixed seeds.

Lunch - Vegetable soup, tuna salad with olive oil and lemon dressing.

Mid afternoon snack - Apple, chunk of cheese and a handful of almonds.

Dinner - Brown rice with baked mackerel and stir-fired vegetables.

OR

Breakfast - Bowl of cereal with milk, sliced banana and toasted nuts, fruit juice.

Mid Morning Snack - Skinny latte, fruit and nut bar.

Lunch - Brown bread sandwich with salmon and cucumber, 3 bean salad.

Mid Afternoon Snack - Tray of raw baby vegetables with low fat 'Philly' and a smoothie.

Dinner - Roast chicken with roast vegetables and a drizzle of flax seed oil.

So how does your day look?

It is **very** unlikely that you came up with an exact copy of either of the above daily combinations. In fact, your day may not have included any of the above foods. **BUT THIS IS THE POINT OF THE EXERCISE.** Eating well, choosing wisely and losing fat is **not** about repeating the same breakfasts, lunches, dinners and snacks until you can no longer bear the sight of or crunch your way through another carrot. The possible combinations from these three lists are endless and these are just a selection from the vast range of great foods available to us which means that if there are certain health-giving foods you really can't stomach, there are always alternatives.

That's why a permanent *Fat Loss Plan* which is light on rules works. Flexibility is key because life can seriously get in the way. Many diets fail because they present us with a lengthy shopping list, instruct a clear out of cupboards, fridge and freezer and insist we stock up on all the *worthy* foods we are going to be eating over the next two or three weeks. It's all crystal clear and we know exactly what we are going to be eating next Thursday for dinner (unexciting or what?) But, when a last minute invitation appears or we have to work late or our kids forget to tell us about some extra curricular activity the plan goes flying out the window. One thing is for sure, life rarely goes to plan.

Following a diet to the letter is a great deal more difficult than learning a few basics which enable us to make the best possible choices when the plan goes pear-shaped. So, if there is the slightest whiff of diet boredom or endless repetition, give it a wide berth. Some of us like to pick and choose, others can't function without a list and a few directives. *The Fat Loss Plan of Action* in chapter 13 is about picking and choosing meals and snacks that appeal and fit in with your day, every day, no matter how hectic your timetable. However, if you really want a few rules and a more prescriptive plan to get you into the fat busting zone I recommend you start with the *2 Weeks in the Fast Lane Plan* in chapter 16 before moving on to designing your own personal fat loss eating strategy.

The 'Fat Boy' Wins the Day

As mentioned, many diets champion losing *weight* rather than losing *fat*. When we follow the recommendations religiously we may well lose *10lbs in 10 days* or whatever the promise and our iron will is rewarded when we leap on the scales every morning and watch the pounds disappearing. It's a good feeling. Furthermore, by the end of 10 days we may even manage to fit into those jeans that have been gathering dust at the back of the wardrobe and our friends and family comment on how great we are looking – it's euphoric and we resolve to *stay with the programme* for another 10 days. Sure, we have read or heard that the average amount of fat that can be lost in a week is unlikely to be more than one or two pounds but we reckon our dedication to the task in hand is knocking that theory on the head so we press on with the reduced *whatever* diet in an effort to see even more pounds drop off. Then along comes the *diet plateau*, the day where the scales show no loss of pounds or even worse a gain – how can that be we ask, we haven't deviated from the regime and we have been saint-like in our devotion to bean sprouts? The euphoria dissipates, we confess that we have actually been feeling increasingly tired, the nagging headache won't budge and everybody and everything is annoying us. We dream of chocolate cake and long for a night out with the girls/lads sharing a pizza and a few cocktails/beers. We are hungry goddammit! Hungry for food, hungry for conviviality, hungry for satisfaction – to see, to touch, to hear, to smell and to taste that longed-for burger on the grill and chips in the deep fat fryer.

The crucial point here is that if the body doesn't get sufficient energy from the nutrients supplied by the food we eat at regular intervals during the day, it quickly adapts and steals from wherever there's a quick, easy and ready source of energy and our muscles are all too obliging. We need only look at pictures of starving families in war-torn third world countries where political unrest, drought and famine are all too common for proof. Bloated stomachs and skeletal arms and legs are the norm. Why? Because muscle is an excellent energy storage site of both glycogen (stored glucose) and protein – both of which can be turned into energy when it is in short supply. Muscle can store up to 500gms (around 2000kcals) of glycogen which holds around **three times** that amount of water. So, if we restrict our food intake dramatically the body gets energy from the stored glycogen in the muscles and water is released along with it. Result - 4lbs lost in 24 hours. Exactly the quick weight loss we were looking for. Continuing with the restrictive regime, the body starts to convert the protein in the muscles into energy and it holds around **four times** its weight in water so even more pounds are lost and we become hooked on that morning ritual of stepping on the scales and congratulating ourselves on yet another couple of pounds lost.

But is the goal to lose 4lbs of fat or 4lbs of precious muscle and a few litres of water? And, as soon as we start eating normally again the glycogen stores are replaced and **so is the water** and we regain some or all of the weight lost and its back to square one. Worse still, instead of re-stocking the hungry muscles, much of the food is turned into fat because the body has become used to *famine mode* and in an effort to store energy wherever possible it becomes increasingly efficient at turning food into fat - it's all about survival. So instead of the lean look we were striving for we end up with weak skinny muscles and a return of the muffin top. A depressing situation, but once we get to grips with this biochemical reality, the pressure is off.

We can start eating to lose fat, rather than starving to gain weight.

There are a number of reasons why many diets don't work. Or more accurately, work initially, enabling many to lose pounds if not stones in a matter of weeks or months only to see some or all of it piling back on as soon as they decide they have reached their target weight or can't cope with the deprivation any longer. One reason is that the body is pre-programmed to survive under the most deprived conditions and when energy from food is restricted it goes into *preservation mode* by slowing down the rate at which food is converted into fuel and hanging onto precious fat stores for what it perceives as the *famine* ahead. Not exactly what we want when we are struggling to shed weight and shift those love handles. If the human body didn't have the ability to press the *preservation button* we wouldn't be here today to discuss.

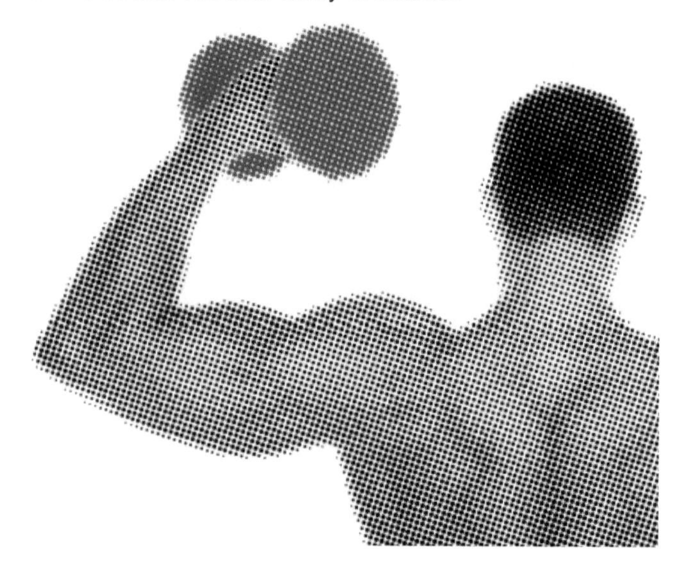

An abundance of food is a relatively recent thing; our ancestors would have given their right arm to have the choices we now have. We didn't always have the luxury of deciding between the blueberry and the banana or the *takeaway* and the *sit in*. If you could gather it or kill it, you took it home and gorged on every morsel, knowing that tomorrow may bring another day of sharing a few roots, berries and leaves between the entire family. One reason we have made it to the 21st century is because of our ability to slow down the metabolism of available nutrients and keep us functioning until the next time food becomes available. Throughout history the man with the most fat stores was invariably the one who survived - famine, war, drought, destitution and torture didn't wipe him out because his body adapted. The skinny ones often didn't make it – no fat stores meant fewer nutrients and death more often than not. Of course it's all very different in the Western world now where food is abundant, but the 21st century body hasn't quite caught up with this situation – it still sees a lack of nutrients as a threat and reacts accordingly. It continues to slow down metabolism in an effort to hang onto nutrients to keep us alive.

Another reason many diets don't work is that our eating patterns are largely controlled by our brain which is constantly adapting to physical and emotional situations and demands fuel 24/7.

We no longer eat just because we are hungry – oh, that it were so simple.

Hunger is quickly recognised by the brain and the message comes through loud and clear "eat something to stop the stomach rumblings, cope with the energy dip and sharpen the fuzzy brain". But, while the brain recognises hunger, it doesn't tell us what to eat to satisfy the hunger. It doesn't say "eat the tuna salad which will not only fill you up but also provide the nutrients to keep you firing on all cylinders for the next few hours and body-swerve the chocolate cake which could see you reaching for another slice within the hour". No, we are left with that unenviable decision and that's where desire comes in. Of course we know that the tuna salad is the healthier option but sometimes the chocolate cake refuses to take a back seat. But hey, the brain's happy, at least for now, we're happy because that sugary, fatty combination provides a load of pleasurable feelings and hunger is satisfied. However, we are all too aware that chocolate cake is never likely to play a big part in the diet we are trying to stick to and before long negativity starts to creep in and we beat ourselves up for giving in to desire and weak will. We then do one of two things. We either give ourselves a thoroughly good talking to and resolve to be a great deal stricter and follow the programme to the letter or we give up, deciding that this diet is obviously not the one. But, before long we embark on another hoping this time we have found the answer.

Giving in to desires and being weak-willed is only a very small part of the equation. Survey upon survey of failed dieters reveal that most blame their failure to lose fat or maintain initial fat loss on their inability to stick to a diet which is depressing for dieters globally but manna from heaven for the dieting industry. Understanding why fat is stored so efficiently and how we can give fat cells a proverbial *kick up the ass* to get them to release energy and shrink is the secret to success and a big breakthrough for many.

Food is Fuel

Fuel is vital for functioning and fat burning

The comparison of the car to the body is perhaps overly simple but is a good place to start. Without fuel the car won't go, without fuel the body won't function or more accurately, won't function too well. The food we eat provides the essential nutrients we need for energy, growth, repair and regeneration, protection and fat burning. A shortage of any results in one, two or possibly all of these processes being compromised over time. The word essential is where many get confused. We cannot expect the body to perform these vital functions if we don't give it the essentials. Carbohydrates, proteins, fats, vitamins, minerals and water are *The Big 6* and we need the lot. What they are, where we find them, when we should eat them and how we should combine them are all covered in the next chapter, *A Little Knowledge is not a Dangerous Thing* and in chapter 13, *The Fat Loss Plan of Action* but don't skip to them yet as there are a few more nuggets to digest which may prove invaluable.

Restriction of the essentials doesn't go unnoticed by the body. It copes in the short term, drawing the missing nutrients from stores but after a while messages are sent to the brain to say "where are the B vitamins, we're running short" or "for Christ's sake give us some carbohydrates" and hunger takes over. We fight it for a time but sooner or later it becomes so strong that it needs to be satisfied, so we hit the starchy, sugary foods with a vengeance. The same applies to low-ANYTHING diets. It's not merely about lack of willpower or self-discipline; it's the body's cry for help and nourishment.

Many reveal that when they are *on* a diet their energy levels take a serious nose dive. Hardly surprising when they are possibly short on the nutrients required to create energy. Also, when we lack energy we feel less inclined to be physically active and when we are less physically active the body doesn't have to call on the fat stores to provide energy – catch 22. Furthermore, many experience mood swings, lack of concentration, confusion, forgetfulness, feel the cold more acutely and their *get up and go* has *got up and gone*. Under these circumstances it becomes increasingly hard to focus on the goal and every day becomes a battle between the body, the brain and the diet and it's no fun. What began as a challenge quickly turns into a war – and guess who's likely to win?

Part 2. Chapter Six

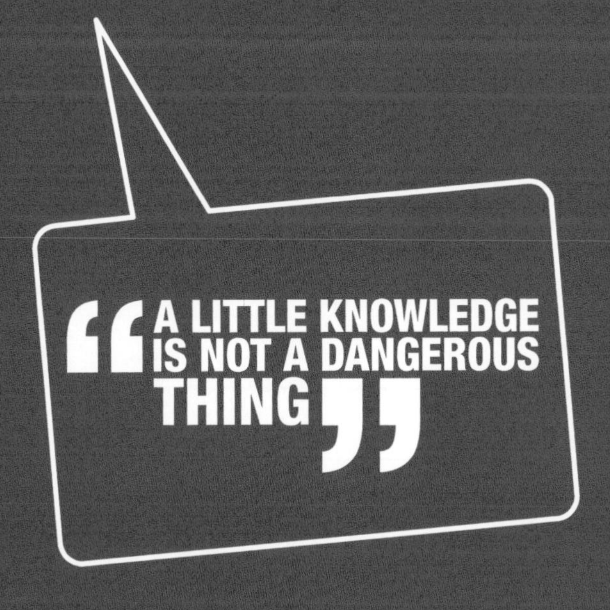

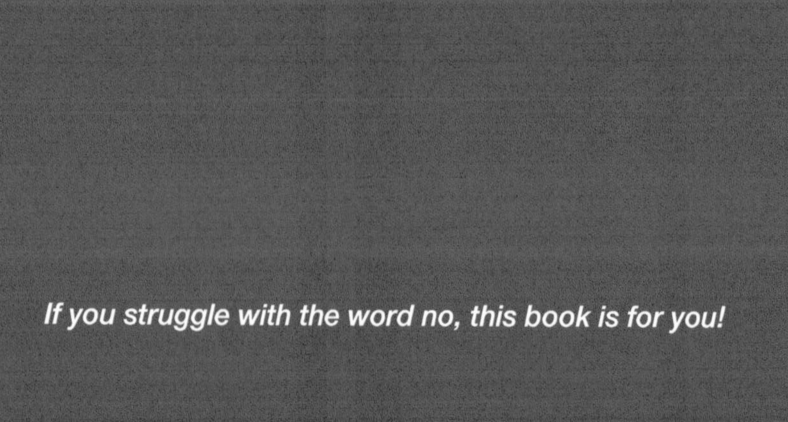
If you struggle with the word no, this book is for you!

Frustratingly, food is now split into two camps. It is either good for us or bad for us. Why this has happened is difficult to fathom but if the intention is to provide us with the information we need to make predominantly *good choices* it's not working. Many of us are more confused than ever! When we understand how foods are processed and used by the body we can evaluate which ones are most likely to work on a personal level, improve our health and promote fat loss, but when we are being bombarded with conflicting messages it can be very hard to find a workable route. What we want is a little knowledge, not information overload. Taking time to digest just a few 'basics' gives us that knowledge. A healthy diet that promotes fat loss can be painless or tortuous dependent on the choices we make but when we know why some foods provide us with energy and nourishment while others provide little other than short term satisfaction, success is a lot more likely.

Every cell in the body works around the clock. There are no weekends off, holidays or duvet days. They just keep going day after day from the moment we are born until the moment we breathe our last doing the very best they can to keep us functioning on all levels. As long as our diet provides them with the right nutrients, they deliver. But they do have preferences and the better the feed, the more efficient. Body cells don't go on strike when they are not getting '5 a day' or being asked to thrive on water and the occasional apple but they do send a red alert to the brain saying "nourishment please" and some cells may be forced to give up nutrient stores they can ill-afford to part with. So how do we ensure that they are all happy and healthy? By understanding where the nourishment comes from.

Fats

Next to water which makes up around 70% of our total weight, fat is the most abundant substance found in the body. Every cell has an outer layer of fat which not only provides protection but also allows the efficient transportation of nutrients in and waste out through the cell membranes – the important layers of tissue that separate the inside of the cells from their outside environment. Furthermore, fat provides a cushion around organs and joints, enhances nerve transmission and keeps skin looking plump and wrinkle-free (well, for a while anyway!)

Around 60% of the brain is fat and without it communication of thoughts, feelings and reactions as well as our interpretation and sense of everything around us is impaired. Fat also ensures hormones stay in prime condition, particularly sex hormones. Fat is truly our friend and ally for energy, fitness, fat loss, heart health, immunity, procreation and longevity. But which fats should we eat?

It's a complicated subject but in an effort to cut through the confusion, we can split the foods rich in fats into four camps.

1. Those that must be included in our diet because we can't make them within the body but they are essential for the above functions.
2. Those that are not essential for the above functions but offer other health benefits.
3. Those that we don't need to include in our diet as we can make them within the body and when eaten in small quantities offer some health benefits.
4. Those that should be avoided as they do us no favours health-wise.

Group one includes most seeds and nuts and their oils and butters, oily fish, soya beans and tofu, group two includes olives, avocados, peanuts and their oil, beans, lentils, chickpeas, eggs and green leafy vegetables and group three includes lean meat, poultry, game and low fat dairy products. Group four is the real danger zone. Trans fats, hydrogenated fats and semi-hydrogenated fats are fats that started out as health-giving oils derived from plants but have been altered and subjected to a dizzying array of chemical processes to manufacture them more cheaply and give them a longer shelf life. They offer little nutritional benefit to the body and when consumed regularly interfere with the metabolism of the fats in the other three groups, reducing their effectiveness and increasing the risk of inflammation within the body which can, over time compromise health. Sadly, these altered fats give foods the kind of fatty taste that makes us want to eat more of them and are present in many processed and fast foods and most junk foods.

The good news is that they have to be itemised on food labels so look out for them and avoid them where possible. Most of the vegetable oils bottled in clear plastic containers that line supermarket shelves should also be viewed with suspicion – the fact that they are being sold at knock-down prices is usually an indication that they have been over-processed and contain few if any health-giving fats. Instead, use olive, coconut or avocado oil or a little butter mixed with one of these oils for cooking and use nut and seed oils for drizzling over soups, stews and vegetables after cooking or in dressings, dips and smoothies.

Protein

Protein may only account for about 12% of total body weight but that 12% defines us as living, breathing, standing, moving, thinking and functioning human beings. Proteins are the building blocks of our uniqueness. They are present in every cell and are the chief components of skin, bones, hair, fingernails, muscles and hormones. They also protect us from disease by creating antibodies that fight foreign invaders and transport oxygen from the lungs to body cells to create energy from food. But, what makes us truly unique is our DNA and every cell uses the information encoded in our genes, which is a kind of *protein library* as the blueprint for making the hundreds of thousands of different proteins that give us our uniqueness.

Little, often and varied is the way to go with protein foods. Meat, poultry, game, fish, shellfish, dairy products, eggs, beans, lentils, legumes, nuts, seeds, a few grains and even a couple of vegetables (spinach and broccoli) provide good levels and the cumulative effect of including a mix of protein foods into our daily diet by having one or maybe two small portions with every meal and snack provides a healthy body with what it needs. Don't overdo them however as this can overwork the liver and kidneys but don't forget them. When it comes to fat loss, they not only help slow down the release of glucose into the bloodstream and keep cravings at bay but also keep us feeling fuller for longer.

NB: Processed meats are cured with sugar, salt and rather too many unpronounceable extras so keep them to a minimum.

Carbohydrates

Glucose is the preferred energy source for every living cell, particularly those in the brain and nervous system and carbohydrates provide a super-fast energy delivery service. The speed with which they can be broken down into glucose molecules, released into the bloodstream then, via the liver shuttled off to body cells to provide the tools to create energy gives them their pole position. If some of the glucose derived from the carbohydrates in a meal or snack is not immediately required it is stored in the liver and muscles as glycogen and when the energy factories within every body cell (the mitochondria) call for more, the glycogen is quickly converted back into glucose, released into the bloodstream and delivered accordingly. It's an efficient system which demands respect.

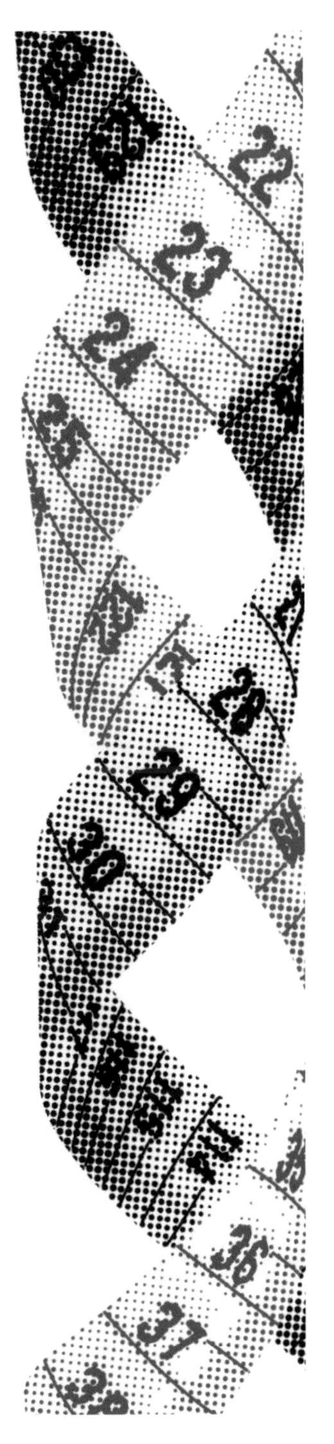

Low carbohydrate diets have become a big hit with dieters because quick weight loss results for many but current lifestyles are demanding and energy requirements are high so we need the super-fast energy that carbohydrate-rich foods provide. Plus, they provide fibre. Without fibre in our diet we are looking at blood sugar swings that can turn us from angels into witches in a matter of hours, digestive problems that can go from being mildly inconvenient to debilitating over time and a proliferation of unfriendly bacteria in the gut which produce toxins that weaken our immune system.

Carbohydrates generally get labelled as *good* or *bad* more often than the other food groups, chiefly because refined grains predominate in the Western diet. In their natural state, grains have a protective outer coating rich in micronutrients which protects them from the environment and disease. When we eat unprocessed grains we benefit from these protective micronutrients but refining removes the outer coating and along with it the micronutrients. They are quick and easy to digest which makes them popular with the consumer and they can be used to produce a wealth of inexpensive foodstuffs making them popular with manufacturers but they are a poor substitute for the real thing. Eating a rainbow of colours is the best way to get maximum nourishment from carbohydrates. Fruits, vegetables, grains, beans, lentils, legumes, nuts and seeds are tops.

If it is white it has been robbed of nutrients and should be regarded as an occasional player rather than a regular fixture in our diet.

Only when we consume a combination of fats, proteins and carbohydrates can we hope to look good, feel great and shed fat and each one of these three macronutrients plays a crucial role in the body. Drastically reducing any of them or worse still cutting one out is madness and forces the body to readjust, which it may cope with in the short term but not in the long term. Macronutrient deficiencies lead to less efficient metabolism of the food we eat and less effective fat burning.

Enzymes

The pace and efficiency of the digestive process has a major influence on the pace and efficiency of the delivery of nutrients to body cells. Metabolism is the series of chemical reactions that make it all happen and enzymes are the catalysts (biochemical spark plugs) that facilitate these reactions. Enzymes are sometimes referred to as our *life force* because we would not exist without them. They are just some of the proteins that are created from the amino acids that form the component parts of the protein foods we eat - yet another reason why protein is so important in our diet. Cells take energy from food during the metabolic process with the help of enzymes but these enzymes need *coenzymes* and *cofactors* to get the job done and that's where vitamins and minerals come in. They are classified as micronutrients because we only need micro amounts to facilitate the metabolism of foods and initiate and assist in the myriad of biochemical processes which sustain life. When our diet is deficient in any or many of these *micro magicians* we are looking at an impaired or poor biochemical performance and the possibility of diminishing health and immunity. Why risk it?

But how do you ensure that you are getting the full package of vitamins and minerals into your daily diet without spending time you probably can't spare analysing the vitamin and mineral content of the foods you eat? Answer - go for variety, experiment whenever possible and above all, make both your life and your food colourful. Vitamins and minerals must be obtained from our diet either because the body can't make them or can't make them in sufficient amounts so it's up to us to get them on board through the food choices we make.

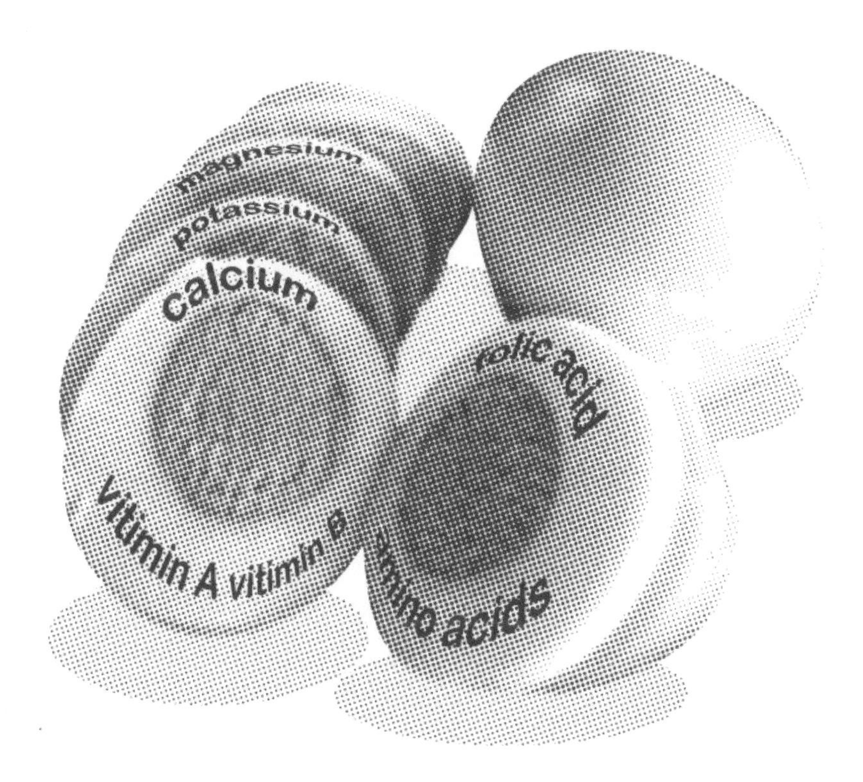

Most low calorie and very low calorie diets don't provide enough micronutrients and if enzymes are short of helpers they can't keep the metabolic fire burning efficiently and post-diet weight gain is likely. *The Fat Loss Plan* in this book ensures you won't be short-changed and avoids this counterproductive and frustrating *metabolic meltdown*.

The Other Essential is Water

If enzymes are the *life force*, then water is the *river of life*. We can't live for more than four or five days without it and as mentioned around 70% of the body is water. It transports nutrients in and waste out of the cells, carries waste from the body and helps maintain body temperature. It has been suggested that drinking more water can increase our metabolic rate and burn more calories but there is scant evidence to support this theory. But, it is important to remember that whilst the enzymes which make everything happen require vitamins and minerals to get the job done, water is the stuff that allows the reactions to take place and ensures that nutrients from food are digested, absorbed and metabolised.

Some people worry that drinking too much water causes fluid retention and may thwart their weight loss goal. Not so. Water retention can occur as a result of certain health problems but from a nutritional point of view it is often as a direct result of having too much or too little salt in the body which upsets the balance between sodium and potassium. How to ensure a good balance of these vital minerals is discussed later in the book.

Probably the most talked about and successful way in which increasing water consumption can help to bust fat is due to the fact that we sometimes mistake thirst for hunger and reach for food when water is possibly what the body is looking for. Additionally, when dieters replace their daily drinks (fizzy drinks and alcohol to name two of the worst culprits) with water, consumption of sugar takes a major dive and that is one great gift we can give ourselves when fat loss is the goal.

Recommendations and tips on how to get a good balance of all of the above and keep the metabolic fire burning all day, every day are included in *The Fat Loss Plan* in chapter 13.

Metabolic Madness

Is yours fast or slow? Can you boost it or quell it? Can an extra chilli in your curry really make a difference or should you just wear less clothes and turn down the thermostat to keep the *fat burning furnace* firing?

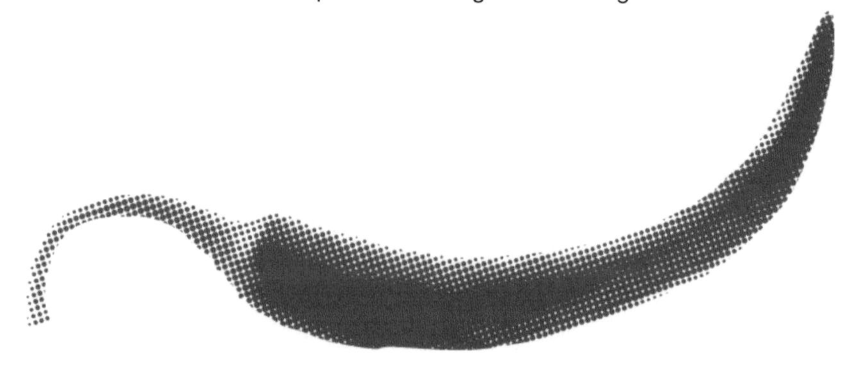

Boosting metabolism to lose weight is currently the *hot ticket* and there's no shortage of advice. As ever, numbers appear to play a major role:- "12 Ways to Revive and Boost Your Metabolism", "15 Best Foods to Boost Your Metabolism", "8 Metabolism Boosters to Help You Burn Fat" etc. Increasing the amount and type of exercise we do on a daily basis is generally involved somewhere along the line, although there are quite a few programmes that somewhat simplistically suggest that merely adding grapefruit, yoghurt, almonds or green tea to our diet does the trick!

Metabolism is a complicated chemical process, so it's no surprise that many people think of it in its simplest sense: as something that influences how easily the body gains or loses weight. Our BMR (basal metabolic rate) is a measure of the rate at which we burn energy in the form of calories while at rest. This can play a role in our tendency to gain or lose weight. For example, a person with a low BMR will tend to gain more pounds of body fat over time compared with a similar-sized person with an average BMR who eats the same amount of food and gets the same amount of exercise. To a certain extent our BMR is inherited and sometimes health problems can affect it but we can turn it up a notch or two. Increasing our level of exercise can not only prompt the body to burn more calories directly from the activity itself but becoming more physically fit can increase the rate. Our BMR is also influenced by body composition and people with more muscle and less fat generally have higher BMRs. This is why, unfairly men gain weight more slowly than women – they have more muscle. But are there certain foods or combinations of foods that can boost the basal metabolic rate?

Thermogenesis

Thermogenesis is the production of heat by the cells within the body. It creates a situation whereby the mitochondria (energy factories) in fat and muscle tissue produce heat instead of energy. Body temperature increases, creating a feeling of warmth, fat is used for fuel and calories are burned. Shivering is the fastest thermogenic process in the body creating heat in super-quick time which can be life-saving in certain circumstances, exercise comes a close second but it is the role that food plays in thermogenesis that has sparked interest and a great deal of research in recent years in the race to find the diet that could halt growing obesity levels.

When we have just eaten, our body temperature automatically rises as energy is created to metabolise the food but it's not significant. The possibility that there may be foods that could raise it further and encourage more fat to be used for fuel is tantalising not only to scientists but also to dieters. Thus far results are confusing and contradictory. Despite the lengthy lists we may come across of *foods guaranteed to increase fat burning* there is actually only one substance that has proven itself to be a real thermogen and that's *capsiate* which is found in chillies but sadly we have to eat rather a lot of them to get the thermogenic effect and because most chillies are much richer in *capsaicin*, the substance that gives them their intense heat this may present a few problems for most of us. However, scientists have created a new variety of sweet pepper called *CH-19* which doesn't contain *capsaicin* but is rich in *capsiate*. We could see these taking centre stage in the vegetable section fairly soon so look out for them.

The Science of Food

When you open your paper in the morning and see an alarming headline like "Calories in Iced Coffee Increase Your Risk of Cancer", how do you react? Dismay, distress, disbelieve or just confusion?

The sharp consumer takes a few minutes to evaluate the study being quoted. Was it an animal or a human study and if it was human how many people were involved? Was it an intervention study or an epidemiological study and did the results contradict previous research? Here's a short explanation of the four different types of studies food researchers undertake which may help to cut through at least some of the confusion:-

Lab Studies

These are generally performed on rats that can be dissected after the study, unlike humans. Being able to use a particular breed ensures that there is a similar physiology which gives scientists greater control over the study. They can also use as many subjects as budget allows and the more there are the more valid the results are likely to be. Humans don't come in breeds however and whilst our physiology is similar to a degree it can't be proven without doubt that similar findings would result. The same applies to test tubes (*in vitro* studies).

Individual Case Studies

These focus on a person or persons who have shown some sort of unusual resistance to disease or have responded in an unexpected way to certain foods or dietary practices. Like the person who ate nothing but baked beans for a year but didn't appear to be nutritionally deficient or the man who ate a dozen eggs a week but whose cholesterol levels were that of a person half his age. Many of these are anecdotal but the ones that make it into the scientific journals can certainly lead to further research. However, a single case study is not regarded as significant proof.

Population Studies

Also known as epidemiological studies. These include studies such as the *Seven Countries Study* which was initiated by American nutritionist, Ancel Keys and looked at the relationship between diet and coronary disease in men in the US, Finland, the Netherlands, Italy, the former Yugoslavia, Greece and Japan. It involved nearly 12,000 people and was recorded over 15 years and resulted in the *Mediterranean-Style* diet being associated with a lower risk of heart disease. These studies are regarded as being statistical and generally uncover a possible connection between diet and disease but don't always allow for the finer details of exact diet composition or lifestyle factors. They do however lay the groundwork for further study.

Clinical Studies

Also known as intervention studies. This is where one group of people receive treatment/nutrients and another group receive a *placebo* and neither the researchers nor the participants know which is which. This type of study takes time and money but can reveal excellent and provable results. But as with ALL studies, the results have to be proven many times over before they are accepted.

You may wish to do more of your own research about the latest studies before you leap into the unknown (some reliable resources are suggested at the back of the book) but it is vital to remember that many are funded by industries who have a vested interest in proving the health-enhancing properties of their products and are more than a little enthusiastic about *feeding their findings to the media*. Don't believe everything you read, employ a degree of scepticism and if you can, stick to fresh, colourful foods 80% of the time and treat the rest as occasional players. You may wish to log on to Ben Goldacre's *Bad Science* website *www.badscience.com* - he certainly doesn't pull any punches when it comes to unveiling those that he believes use bogus scientific research to make claims (and he's none too fond of nutritional therapists either!)

Part 2. Chapter Seven

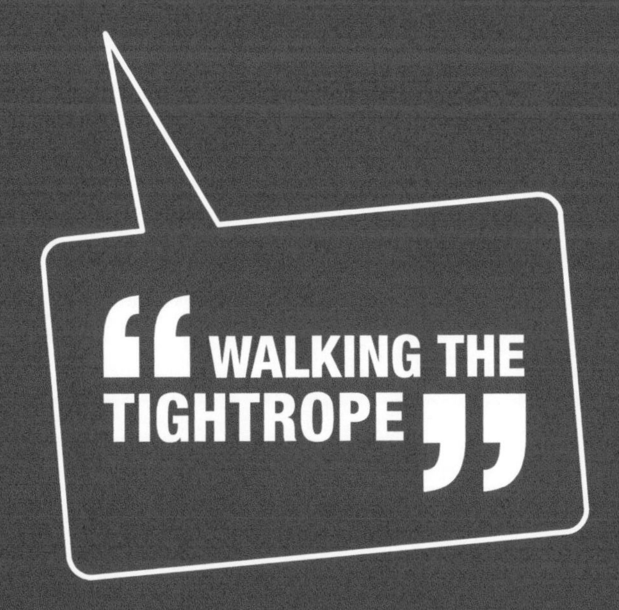

Protein makes us truly unique and unique is good!

Are you confused about the blood sugar thing? You are not alone!

For some people, understanding the principles behind blood sugar highs and lows is absolutely vital. Type 1 diabetics must know exactly how to monitor blood glucose levels as failure to do so can result in serious health complications. This condition requires understanding, compliance and regular medication or insulin therapy. Similarly, those who have been diagnosed with Type 2 diabetes are professionally advised on how to manage their blood sugar. Hypoglycaemia (recurring episodes of low blood sugar) can be a precursor to Type 2 diabetes and should not be ignored. If there is a history of this condition in your family or you are experiencing certain symptoms regularly (raging thirst, frequent urination, dizzy spells, blurred vision, inexplicable tiredness, an addiction to sweets) go and see your doctor.

Dysglycaemia, on the other hand is where people lurch roller-coaster style from blood sugar highs to blood sugar lows throughout the day and sometimes during the night and these are generally exaggerated by what and when we eat. Getting off the roller-coaster is important and managing the release of the hormones insulin and glucagon into the bloodstream has to be addressed in order to prevent the sort of blood sugar havoc that can lead to fatigue, mood swings, low energy levels and a myriad of other symptoms.

Too much of ANYTHING in the bloodstream at any one time, be it sugar, calcium, fats, salt or toxins sets off alarm bells and the body moves into overdrive to restore balance by removing any excess.

When it comes to glucose in the bloodstream, around one to three teaspoons is acceptable but any more and the pancreas leaps into action to assist in its removal - this is damage limitation at its best.

In an ideal situation the levels of insulin and glucagon are counterbalanced in the bloodstream. Just after eating a meal or snack, the body is primed to take delivery of the glucose from carbohydrate foods, fatty acids from fats and amino acids from protein foods. The presence of these substances in the intestine stimulates the pancreas to release the hormone, insulin into the bloodstream and rise. This prompts cells, particularly liver, fat and muscle cells to absorb the incoming molecules of glucose, fatty acids and amino acids and ensures that the concentration of glucose doesn't rise dangerously high. In contrast, between meals or when we are asleep, the cells continue to need supplies of glucose in order to keep functioning. Slight drops in blood glucose levels stimulate the secretion of the hormone, glucagon from the pancreas. Glucagon prompts the liver and muscles to break down stored glycogen and release glucose into the bloodstream and also prompts the liver and kidneys to produce and release glucose from amino acids and the glycerol part of fatty acids ensuring that the concentration of glucose doesn't fall dangerously low. The interplay between insulin and glucagon secretions throughout the day and night help keep the blood glucose concentration constant.

Type 2 diabetes is not caused simply by eating too much sugar.

It is a disease that affects the body's ability to use the glucose poured into the bloodstream after we eat. It is caused by how well or how badly insulin, and to an extent glucagon do their jobs as outlined above. Either the system that signals the pancreas to produce these hormones becomes less efficient over time or body tissues become less responsive to their actions. So why do some of us become insulin-resistant and how can this debilitating condition be avoided?

Being overweight presents one of the greatest risks so getting consumption of sugar under control is an important element in the pursuit of a healthy pancreas and receptive body cells. The wealth of sugars that flood the system as a result of the breakdown of refined carbohydrates plus the vast array of sugars added to many processed foods encourage continued blood sugar fluctuations. The natural sugars in fruits, vegetables, whole grains, pulses, nuts and seeds don't have as dramatic an effect. Additionally, when protein foods and/or a little fat are eaten alongside natural sugars the delivery of glucose into the bloodstream is slower and more steady, the pancreas releases insulin and glucagon as and when required and blood sugar highs and lows are generally avoided. Repeated consumption of refined grains, sugary drinks, sweets and snacks not only lead to weight gain but can also create chaos because the pancreas is continually being called upon to redress the balance and can, ultimately become exhausted. Blood glucose concentration must be kept within safe limits.

So how do you ensure that you don't ask too much of the pancreas but still eat a diet rich in energy-giving carbohydrate foods? By learning to recognise the foods and drinks that are loaded with what are generally regarded as quick-releasing sugars and whilst enjoying them occasionally, knowing when and how to eat them so that the roller-coaster ride doesn't spiral out of control. But they are everywhere! How to spot them is covered in the next chapter *If it Tastes Great it Must be Bad for You.*

Is blood sugar management the single most important thing you need to grasp in order to lose fat?

Not necessarily. It largely depends on your current diet. If you know you are living most days on fizzy drinks, sugary cereals, cakes, biscuits, crisps, takeaways and copious amounts of booze, you are probably also aware that this kind of *road accident* of a diet needs improvement. Keeping the concentration of glucose in the bloodstream constant can be difficult to achieve just as accepting that the complex subject of blood sugar management can be confusing to say the least. The debate about which carbohydrates we should eat, how many and how often continues, but finding a balance that works personally is central to permanent fat loss. Just as we can't expect to make a perfect omelette without a good pan and fresh eggs, we can't expect body cells to create energy without the sugars derived from food – we just have to make sure it's the right kind of sugar!

So, are carbohydrates the enemy in the fat loss game?

Most foods contain a mixture of carbohydrates, protein and fat but some are richer in one than another. Those that contain predominantly carbohydrates include grains, starchy vegetables, fruits, beans and pulses. Non-starchy vegetables also contain carbohydrates but in much smaller amounts than their starchy counterparts. Carbohydrates are built of sugar molecules and come in all shapes and sizes. They are broken down by the body into glucose molecules which circulate in the bloodstream supplying cells with fuel on an as-needed basis. As discussed, any glucose that is not immediately required is converted into glycogen and stored in the liver and muscles and when they are brim full the remainder gets converted into fat and we know where that gets stored - the hips, the thighs, the waistline etc. A call from body cells for more energy prompts the conversion of stored glycogen to glucose which is quickly and efficiently utilised to meet demand. But how do you prompt fat cells to release their stores, which is what you are ultimately looking for when you want to shed fat and become lean?

If the liver and muscles are storing sufficient glycogen to meet energy requirements fat cells remain comfortably idle and untroubled - their stores are not needed. Whilst body cells demand the super-fast energy that carbohydrates provide to feed their glucose requirements and avoid energy dips they rarely differentiate between the carbohydrates that provide longer-lasting energy and those that provide a quick fix. As far as a body cell is concerned there is no such thing as a *bad* carbohydrate - all carbohydrates provide glucose and all carbohydrates can be used to create energy. Some provide a wealth of nutrients, others bring little else to the party other than short-lived energy. Yet again, you have to make the all-important decision as to which ones you consume.

Sugars that naturally occur in foods are important energy-givers, refined and added sugars are weight-gainers - sounds simple because it is. Keeping a watchful eye on where sugars are lurking allows us to gorge on the greats and go easy on the losers. The *low carb* life where fruits, vegetables, whole grains and pulses are put on the back burner makes no sense – super-quick weight loss in super-quick time may be achieved by following this kind of regime but two things are likely to occur within a few weeks. One, cravings for these foods are inevitable because certain vitamins and minerals are missing and as discussed the enzymes needed to get energy from food won't do a very good job without the coenzymes provided by vitamins and minerals. Secondly, where's the fibre? There has never been, and probably never will be a successful long term fat loss success story that ignores the power of fibrous foods. Fibre slows digestion, makes us feel fuller for longer, sweeps through the digestive tract taking with it all sorts of toxins and waste and encourages the growth of healthy bacteria within the colon preventing the unfriendly lot from multiplying and reducing our ability to fight off disease. Additionally, a diet rich in fibrous sugar-rich carbohydrates helps to create a platform whereby the pancreas can produce the all-important blood sugar hormones when required without becoming over-stressed and calling for time out.

So how do you spot the 'roller-coaster' signs?

Here are a few symptoms you may be familiar with:-

- You get a shaky feeling.
- You experience little dizzy spells when you stand up quickly.
- You have blurry vision from time to time.
- You're get fidgety and anxious.
- You could often *kill* for a quick snooze.
- You just can't concentrate on the job in hand.
- You feel you need to eat something but you don't know what.
- Your heart is racing and your breathing is shallow.
- You have a nagging headache you just can't shake.
- You are in a meeting or driving and your eyelids are heavy, heavy, heavy.
- You feel chilled and can't get warm.
- You are listening to someone but the brain fog won't let you take in what they're saying.
- You are more irritable and impatient than normal.

Some of these symptoms may be the result of other health issues but most are a sure sign that blood sugar levels are all over the place. And when this happens the body is more likely to store fat than burn it. Sad but true. The message sent from the body cells to the brain is invariably the same when energy is required "more glucose please, and fast". Then what happens? More often than not we reach for crisps, biscuits, cakes, fizzy drinks or alcohol to provide a quick burst of much-needed energy. The natural sugars in fruits, vegetables and whole grains somehow don't hit the spot. And the tuna salad doesn't get a look in!

Learning to recognise the symptoms that lead us down this path, working out when the roller-coaster is getting out of control and being ahead of the game is a great fat loss strategy. It involves a little planning and can take time out of a busy schedule for a week or so but once we know when our personal energy dips occur we can beat them - it's like finding the pot of gold at the end of the rainbow. There is a whole chapter in part three dedicated to what to keep in the fridge, freezer, desk drawer, handbag, briefcase, glove compartment etc. to make sure you have foods to hand which can control blood sugar swings and tame the devil woman/man within.

Could thinking be making you fat?

Anyone who has ever gone *on* a diet knows only too well where it can all go horribly wrong. You are absolutely determined to stick this one out, you know which foods you should be eating to make it work, you may even have got to grips with a few of the biochemical reasons behind why you may have piled on the pounds. But somehow or other you can't get through another day without giving in to temptation. Then it's back on the slippery slope to diet failure. It's just too hard to stay on the straight and narrow and the only thing you can do is start afresh tomorrow, or next Monday! But who's in charge – your stomach or your brain? Why does temptation keep knocking on the door and foiling your best intentions?

Make no mistake, your brain is in charge and when your brain is hungry it demands to be fed!

It may be only around 2-3% of your body weight but it consumes around 25% of your energy – that's a quarter of the energy you get from food daily just to keep it satisfied. That's one hungry monster! And when it is hungry, it's not

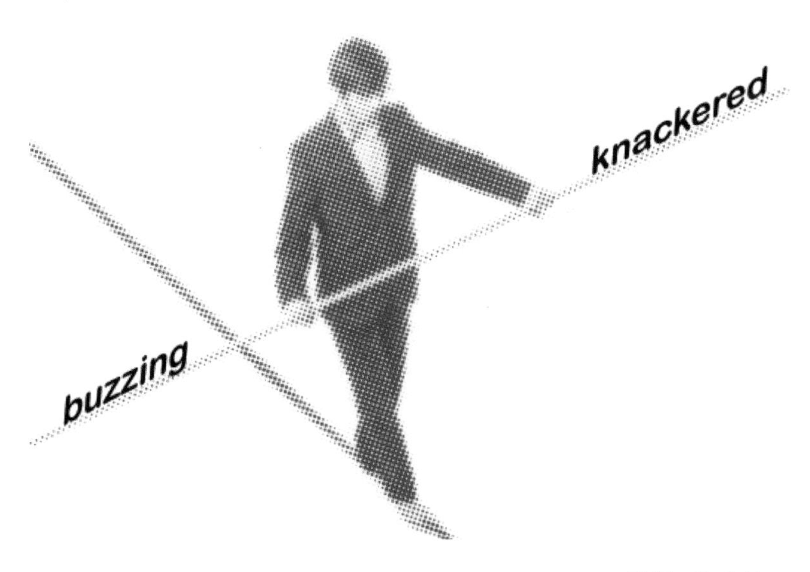

bothered where the energy comes from as long as it comes fast. It is certainly happier, healthier and works a whole lot better if it gets a variety of fabulous foods which provide all the essential nutrients but if a cup of coffee and a pastry is all that is on offer, it will make do - well, at least in the short term.

We think all day and for large chunks of the night and thinking requires energy – energy from food and lots of it. If we are too tired to think, to concentrate, to make decisions or to reason there is a fair chance the brain is hungry. How do we usually feel when a *snack attack* hits? Tired, stressed, blue, confused, worried, bored, frustrated – all negative thoughts and emotions which invariably prompt a desperate need for a *not so good food choice*. When we are feeling positive and upbeat it's much easier to opt for the *good choice* food. When the brain needs to create energy it wants glucose and it wants it now so it immediately calls upon any that is circulating around the bloodstream because the brain takes priority. Once that is scoffed it calls upon the stored glucose in the liver and the muscles. This means that there's less available for other body cells that need to be fed so they go hungry – not an ideal situation as the body can only perform efficiently when it is well fed.

Communication between the brain and the body depends on neurotransmitters and hormones, 'chemical bikers' that work together to relay messages around the body. To keep communication lines open, this vast network has to be fed, regularly and optimally. The brain is an incredible organ. Countless neuroscientists devote their lives to uncovering the intricacies of how best to feed it and there is still a vast amount to learn, but here are the basics:- fats **build** the brain, carbohydrates **fuel** it, micronutrients **protect** it from damage and proteins **unite** the network of neurotransmitters and hormones that communicate with the rest of the body so we have to give it a good balance of all four. Cutting out any of the major food groups or feeding it with too little or too many of any one of them can only result in compromising its health and performance. If we concentrate on feeding the brain, confusion about blood sugar becomes less of an issue.

So how do we keep the brain nutritionally satisfied?

1. **Get it fat – with essential fats**
2. **Give it fuel - with carbohydrates**
3. **Protect it - with micronutrients**
4. **Allow it to communicate - with proteins**

The importance of a good balance of essential fats, carbohydrates, micronutrients and protein for energy, building and repair and defence were covered in the previous chapter but when it comes to brain health, they bear repeating. We cannot expect the brain to do its job, push the boundaries and help us to shed fat if we don't give it the nutrients it needs. So, don't starve it, feed it. Thinking needs the full package of nutrients, so does fat loss.

Part 2. Chapter Eight

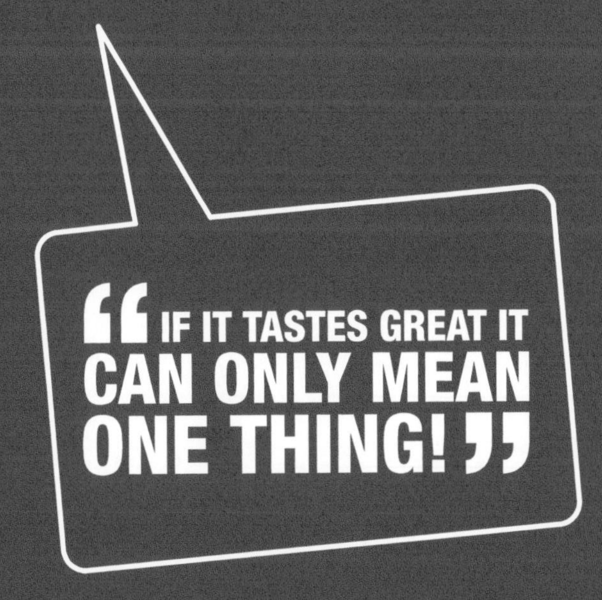

Our ancestors are responsible for our love of sugar, salt and fat-goddamn them!

Sugar, salt and fat make food taste great. But why are they so difficult to resist? Well, it's not our fault. We are hard-wired to love them.

The blame lies with our ancestors because they are responsible for our genetic coding and our love of them. Food was scarce for our ancestors and they ate what they could forage or kill. **Fat** is the most concentrated source of energy and is readily stored so to ensure the continuation of the species, our ancestors ate fat whenever they could to enable them to get through the lean times. Remember, the fat boys invariably outlived the skinnies.

Salt is absolutely vital for controlling the amount of water in the body, maintaining the correct pH of blood, transmitting nerve signals and for muscular contraction. Our ancestors sought out salt or suffered serious consequences, often death.

A sweet tooth allowed them to discern between plants that were safe and those that were deadly – an important skill. They tentatively licked these foods and waited for a reaction, then progressed to a very small bite before ascertaining whether they were nutritious or poisonous. The **sugar** content generally meant they could be eaten and used to nourish them and their children.

It is regularly reported that fat, salt and sugar are bad for us and should be avoided like the plague but this is misleading. They are essential to life and play a major role in a healthy diet and also in successful fat loss. There are a few major problems however; one is that the wrong kinds of fats and sugars take centre stage in the Western diet, two is that salt is either added to a great many products or we load it on to our food to add flavour and three we are simply eating too much of all three. Some think that the blame lies with industrialisation. Sugar, salt and fat which were difficult for our ancestors to find in order to stay alive are now abundant and cheap. It's easy to blame manufacturers for continuing to produce foods that feed our ancestral desire for sugary, salty and fatty foods or be cynical about lacklustre government directives which fail to curb production of foods that feed those desires but we are not being force-fed.

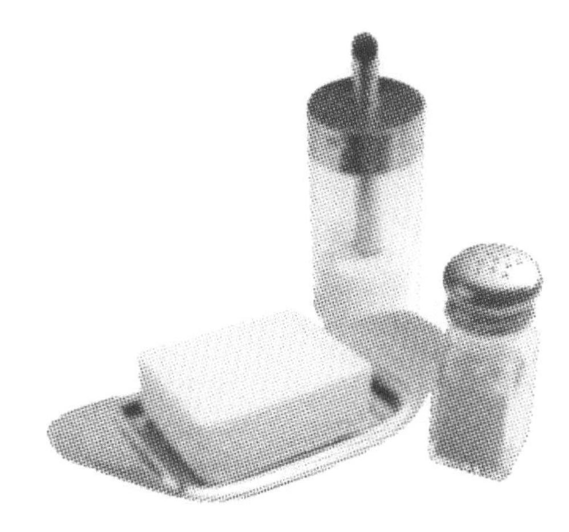

It's up to us to make choices.

Choice can enhance or inhibit our mental and physical health, our earning potential, our ambitions and our enjoyment of life. When we are in charge and not looking to apportion blame elsewhere it is a great deal more satisfying, even when we get it wrong. Dietary choices can be hard mainly because of the confused messages that abound but when we learn a little we know a lot, particularly about what is going to work on a personal level.

The Fat Loss Plan in this book focuses on fresh, unprocessed foods principally because they give us the upper hand nutritionally and we know more or less what we are buying, cooking and eating. But, fast, processed and ready made foods have not been ignored. Time is precious and most of us are forced into opting for convenience occasionally or in some cases regularly. Sadly, many quick and easy meal and snack options are overloaded with refined sugars, salt, saturated fat or all three but there are an increasing number of food companies who work tirelessly to provide us with dishes that are fresh, delicious and nutritionally fab. They are not always the cheapest option because sympathetically-produced food requires time and dedication and when preservatives don't play a part, shelf life is reduced but I urge you to give them a go from time to time - the taste alone speaks volumes.

But, back to the convenience foods that line the supermarket shelves and don't make a dent in your wallet. How do you discern between the good and the not so good? Check out the label. Now, here's a subject that probably causes more confusion than anything discussed so far!

Sugar, salt and saturated fats (the 3 S's) are the ones to watch.

Sugar, Salt + Saturated Fat

Everything is getting sweeter, saltier and fattier and the 3 S's are hidden everywhere. They make foods more palatable and extend their shelf life so you have to be on your guard. Baby foods, breads, burger buns, breakfast cereals, soups, tinned foods, snack foods, pasta sauces, processed cheese, gravies, fruit yoghurts... the list goes on. But it doesn't mean they can't feature on your shopping list. If you know what to look out for they won't invade your life. See later in this chapter for a quick method of spotting the culprits.

Restaurant meals and takeaways present a totally different type of confusion. Menus rarely give details of exactly what goes into their dishes so it is usually a 'best guess' but here's a good trick. If you know there is the likelihood of a ready, fast or restaurant meal at some point in your day when you are unlikely to be able to determine the sugar, salt or saturated fat content, try to ensure you eat fresh, unprocessed foods for the rest of the day – that way you are still in charge of your daily consumption.

The 80:20 Rule

This leads us nicely on to the 80:20 principle. If you get it right 80% of the time you can pretty much do what you like for the other 20%. It works! The 10% of people who make diets work and stay lean for the rest of their lives don't always say no to dessert or body swerve the burger and chips when they are on a night out but they do say no to the 3 S's for the rest of the day. Neither do they starve themselves all day in an effort to keep the calories down to near zero so they can enjoy a few plates of fajitas dripping with cheese and copious cocktails in the evening. Hopefully, the early chapters have made it clear that this kind of starve/binge route is not the way to keep the metabolic fire burning. There is a place for every food in our lives and when we become *metabolically-efficient* by eating the foods that provide us with the kindling to stoke the fire and eat regularly throughout the day, the overly sweet, overly salty and overly fatty foods that are part of our culture can be indulged in occasionally and instead of being dumped as fat can be turned into energy. The 'which, when, where and how' are covered in detail in *The Fat Loss Plan.*

Some people thrive on keeping absolute control of what they eat and don't allow any kind of processed foods into their life and they deserve respect, but most of us have favourites we can't live without which possibly harks back to our ancestral need for sugar, salt and fat. The good news is that total denial of that instinctive drive doesn't have to be on the cards!

But not all fats make us fat

NOT EATING FATS CAN MAKE US FAT. The now well-researched Omega 3 fatty acids already discussed can inhibit fat storage in the body by a rather complex process where they limit the activity of the genes that make the enzymes required for fat production. They also increase thermogenesis, the internal body heat system that accelerates calorie burning. Under the right conditions, Omega 3s and to a lesser extent Omega 6s may prove to have the power to flick a biochemical switch which turns the body from a predominantly carbohydrate-burning machine to a fat-burning machine. Plus, both these essential fatty acids have been shown to make people feel more positive and less depressed which helps to keep dieters focused. Few of us achieve permanent fat loss when negatives invade our day.

Introducing these little nuggets of gold into your life and your diet can make a massive difference. The simple fact is that when we eat foods rich in the Omegas we not only accelerate fat burning but the feeling of fullness they create stems hunger and reduces the cravings that are synonymous with dieting. The added bonus is that Omega 3's in particular, found in oily fish, some nuts, seeds and beans are exceptionally hard to overdose on. Imagine you have just had a *foot long subway* with meatballs and the rest and someone suggests a dessert or ice cream. You are full, but somehow you manage to force it down. Conversely, when you have had a good portion of oily fish and a mixed salad dressed with flax seed oil it is easier to refuse the dessert – you really are stuffed.

These essential fats are essential for our skin, hair, nails, joints, brain and for nerve transmission. If they are doing all that AND helping us to burn fat, they seriously deserve respect. There was a time, around twenty years ago when fats were everything that was bad from a health perspective and the WHO (World Health Organisation) decreed that we should give them a very wide berth. How things change, but that's the wonder of nutritional science and why, if we have the time we should try to keep up to speed. The emerging greatness of essential fats is SO BIG that understanding their role in improving all-round health and perhaps even curbing the global obesity crisis could well take centre stage in the next ten or twenty years. If you would like to know everything there is to know about their amazing health-giving properties just Google 'the fat man' Udo Erasmus – he has spent the last thirty years researching them and if you have a query, he has the answer (link at the back of the book).

Reading the food labels – Aaaagh!

Food is complex stuff, so the first thing to grasp is that we are never going to know exactly how many grams of the 3 S's we are eating in a day unless we cart a load of food tables around with us and look everything up, which can be time consuming to say the least. Also, some food labels are more complicated than they need be, others slip through the net and don't offer sufficient information. However, a few basic pointers allow us to select foods and drinks with a fair degree of confidence.

- Ingredients are listed in order of most, first so if any kind of sugar, salt or saturated fat is near the top it's likely to be a poor choice.
- The more ingredients there are on the label, the greater the likelihood of added sugars and fats so go for foods and drinks with the shortest lists.
- Sugar can be added to a product not only as sugar, but also in many different guises. Anything that ends in *–ose* (glucose, dextrose, maltose etc) is sugar, anything that ends in *–ol* (manitol, sorbitol etc) is sugar in its alcohol form and all syrups are sugar as are caramel, molasses and honey.
- Avoid artificial sweeteners and diet products. A modest amount of table sugar or honey plays a lot less havoc with the body than a bunch of chemicals and they do nothing to lessen sugar cravings.
- Salt can also be listed as *sodium* or *salt equivalent.*
- Look out for trans, hydrogenated or semi hydrogenated fats and oils on the label. These are fats that started life as unsaturated and essential fats but have been chemically altered to extend their shelf life and improve palatability and are found in a great many products. They do us no favours health-wise and should be avoided wherever possible.

Look at the *per 100g* column rather than the *per serving* column and follow these guidelines:-

Spot the Sugar

Where it says *Carbohydrates, of which sugars* 10g is high, 2g is low. Aim for a maximum of 4g.

Spot the Saturated Fat

Where it says *Fats, of which saturates* 5g is high, 1g is low. Aim for a maximum of 2g.

Spot the Salt

Where it says *Salt* or *Salt equivalent* 1.5g is high, 0.3g is low. Aim for a maximum of 0.6g.

Spot the Sodium

Where it says *Sodium* 0.5g is high, 0.1g is low. Aim for a maximum of 0.2g.

And finally, leave the fizzy drinks, fruit squashes and alcopops on the shelf. There are around 10 cubes of sugar in a can of Coca Cola and the rest aren't much better. If they regularly feature in your day you will be amazed at how quickly you can lose fat by just making this one simple change. Even if you choose the *diet* or *zero* versions, they still mess around with your blood sugar and prompt a need for some other sweet treat. Get them out of your life if you can.

Part 2. Chapter Nine

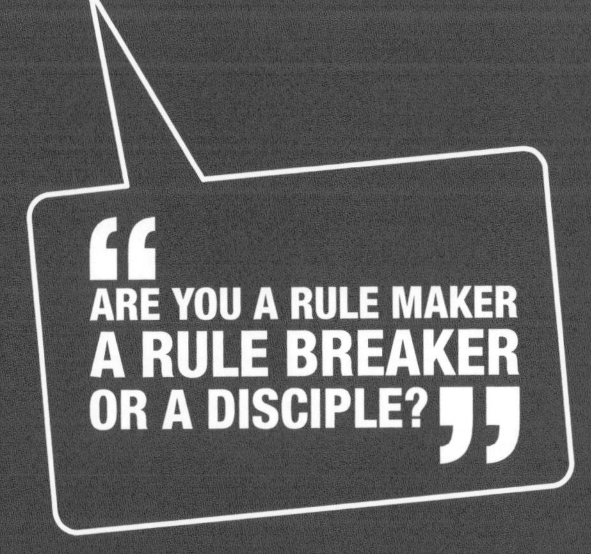

When we know that one or two custard creams often lead to a whole packet we would rather keep that information to ourselves!

There are a number of things that play a major role in whether you get rid of the fat you hate or not and one of them is how you view a diet and exercise programme. You are probably one of the following. You are a rule maker, a rule breaker or a disciple.

If you are a rule maker, you take in every little detail of a diet plan and select only the bits you think will work for you. If you are a rule breaker you read most diet plans with suspicion but embrace some of the basics whilst making a few little alterations. If you are a disciple you are delighted that there is a plan to follow and dive in wholeheartedly. Which works? All of them and none of them! If you are a rule maker you are not overly disappointed when the diet doesn't work because it probably didn't suit your lifestyle so you move on. If you are a rule breaker, you ultimately determine that very little of it made sense so you get back on the search for a more workable alternative. If you are a disciple, you are deeply disappointed because you followed the plan religiously and it let you down.

A very useful trick is to recognise your type. The reason *The Fat Loss Plan* in this book works for many is because you devise a plan that **works for you and your type.** But recognising where your priorities lie is important. A young mum with three small children at home has very different priorities from a single working woman of 30-something. A single man of 32 has very different priorities from a 55 year old executive male with four children and a massive mortgage. Age, views and lifestyle play a big part in the fat loss game. Start by working out whether you are predominantly a rule maker, a rule breaker or a disciple then decide how best to tailor the plan to your life. There could be a bit of all three in you but there is likely one that predominates. *The Fat Loss Plan* offers guidance but only you can decide how best to fit the recommendations into your life. Whatever type you think you are, ask yourself a few difficult, personal questions before you commence. They could help map a route to success.

The reason *The Fat Loss Plan* in this book works for many is because you devise a plan that works for you and your type.

Over the years I have spent a great many hours trying to come up with the ultimate questionnaire to give clients who are determined to lose their 'love handles' or 'man boobs' once and for all. They generally involve questions about how they approach diets, what they find hard about them, which aspects of their lifestyle and family life prevent them from making a few changes to improve their diet, how they feel about exercise etc. but no matter how many times I have tried to convince myself that people like filling in questionnaires and that their answers will enable me to form a picture of where the stumbling blocks may lie, I have ultimately concluded that questionnaires only work when we are not being asked to 'bear our souls'. We all lie and we all answer a percentage of the questions with the answers we think might show us in a better light. We don't mean to be dishonest and we don't go out of our way to be evasive, it's just that when we know that one or two custard creams often lead to a whole packet we would rather keep that information to ourselves! So the questionnaire has been put into a rarely opened file in the documents folder where it is likely to stay. Everybody's story is different and no questionnaire is ever going to allow me to devise a plan that guarantees success. But, what I can do is listen, pinpoint the positives and try to clarify where some of the confusion may lie.

Many practitioners involved in the weight loss game concentrate on uncovering bad habits and whilst they don't physically deliver a slap on the wrist, disapproval is often in the air. By highlighting poor eating practices and suggesting improvements, better habits can be achieved and this method does make some sense both from a fat loss and health perspective, but how many of us want to be reminded that we are falling not just at the first hurdle but at every hurdle! Alterations to eating patterns can only be made when we feel positive and concentrate on what we are doing right, not on what we are doing wrong. Making a list of foods we love (and why) and foods we hate (and why), as recommended in chapter 1 is a good place to start. But we can all dig a little deeper and question why we make certain decisions at certain times. Exposing some of our diet gremlins and deciding whether we like to make our own rules, break a few rules or follow rules to the letter enables us to make a few dietary u-turns.

Rule Makers

Read the book from cover to cover, debate the principles behind every paragraph of every chapter, study *The Fat Loss Plan* and the exercise suggestions then make sure that you adapt the suggestions to fit comfortably into your daily grind and your lifestyle and make it work for you.

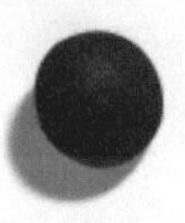

Rule Breakers

Scan the book, flick from back to front and front to back, settle on whichever chapters strike a chord, study *The Fat Loss Plan* and the recommended 'eats', consider how you can change what you keep in your fridge/freezer, briefcase, desk drawer etc and *pik'n'mix* until you find a workable plan. It may take a little time but once you are happy with your choices you won't feel you are playing by the rules.

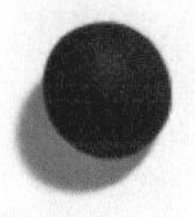

Disciples

This book won't let you down. If you read, understand and digest all that is written and feel empowered to make some changes you can follow the basic guidelines of *The Fat Loss Plan*. What you may find, that differs from many plans you may have followed in the past is that there are few rules. You may want rules however, so start with the *2 Weeks in the Fast Lane Plan* or the *3 Days in the Super-Fast Lane Plan* both of which involve a number of important rules before moving on to design your own dietary strategy which you can stick to for as long as you wish.

What's coming round the corner?

Generally speaking, rule makers and rule breakers have an appetite for what's new and want to hear more about the latest research on fat loss techniques. Disciples are often equally keen. So should we wait for concrete scientific evidence to give us the green light to try out some of the ground breaking musings on how to accelerate fat loss? It all depends on our take on the latest news. Some of us are inquisitive by nature and want to try things out for ourselves before embracing or binning the principles behind them, others simply bin the theory because they suspect it is yet another madcap method of stealing their time and money. It's all about choice. When something becomes a global issue, funds are somehow found and research moves at a pace. Obesity is now a global issue so new ways of tackling it are going to continue to be investigated and new discoveries made that could benefit all. Here's a small selection of the cutting-edge theories you may hear a lot more about in the coming years.

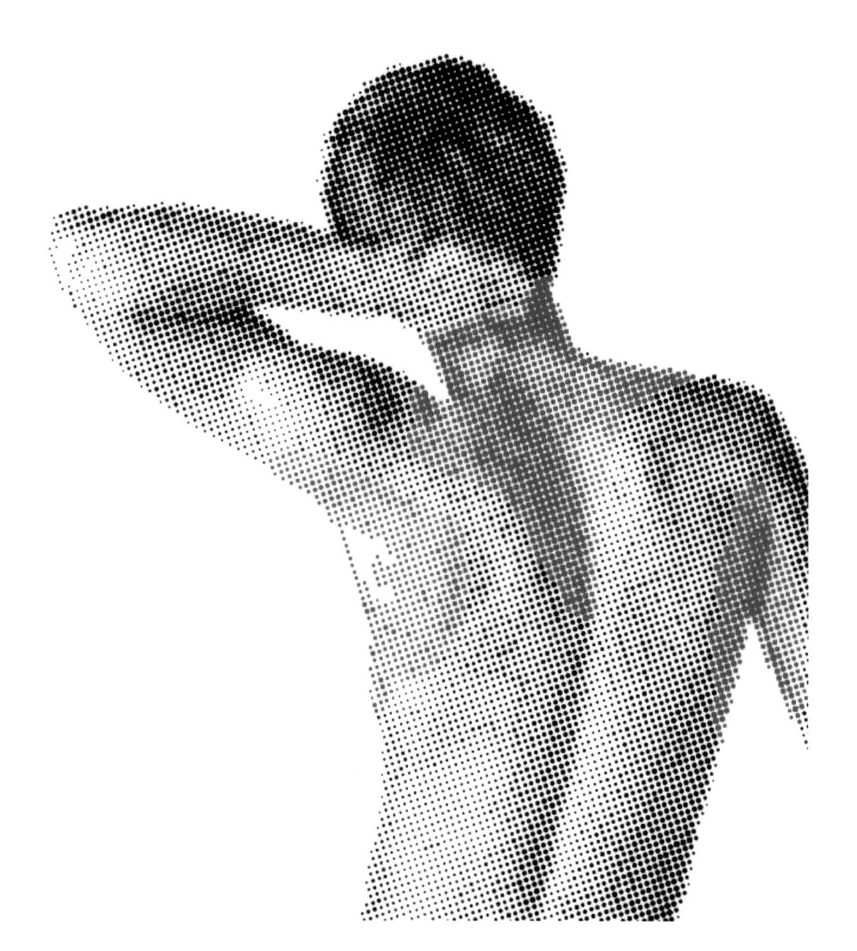

Brown Fat

Most body fat is white fat, the bulky stuff that stores excess calories, makes up cell membranes, insulates nerve cells, cushions our organs and sits on our hips. But we also have small amounts of brown fat and brown fat cells not only have a much richer blood supply but are jam-packed with mitochondria, the energy powerhouses. That makes them a great deal more metabolically active and instead of making energy, they make heat using fat and glucose from the bloodstream for fuel. This means that basal metabolic rate (BMR) increases and more calories are burned. Some estimate that active brown cells can burn up as much as 20% of our daily calorie intake. We are born with a good supply of brown fat cells and as babies we have the ability to turn white fat cells into brown fat cells to keep the body warm but sadly, as we age the process becomes less efficient. However, there is growing evidence that white to brown fat cell conversion can be increased when we are exposed to cold. Taking cold baths and showers, swimming in the cold waters of our British shores or unheated swimming pools, exercising on winter mornings in skimpy shorts and a T-shirt or wearing specially designed clothing that keep the areas that are rich in brown fat cells cool (the armpits and the neck area) have all been investigated. Some of these methods are fairly extreme so unless your health is good, you are advised to consult your doctor before giving them a try.

Other ways of encouraging brown fat cell production and prompting increased calorie burning to keep the body warm may be to turn down the heating thermostat, wear less clothes and sleep in a cool room. If you are over 50 you may remember when the heating only went on in the dead of winter and you always slept in a cold room with the window open - that's when most people were slim so there may be something in it! Read the research to date on brown fat (scientifically known as brown adipose tissue or BAT) – it's fascinating stuff and could hold the key to increased fat burning in the future. Details of cutting-edge (but expensive) clothing products that help to keep the areas where brown fat cells are at a premium cool, are at the back of the book.

Calorie Cycling

Also known as calorie shifting, zig-zag dieting or carbohydrate control. This type of diet has been used successfully over the last ten years or so by natural bodybuilders - those who refuse to use drugs to shed fat fast in the run up to a competition, but it's a real *hot potato* where healthy fat loss is concerned. Few disagree that taking in less calories than we expend in a day is our first port of call when we want to lose weight and keep it off. There is also little dispute about the role of regular exercise, muscle being more metabolically active than fat which makes it an effective calorie burner. There is also universal disrespect for very low calorie diets because if we starve the body of energy, it will turn down the metabolic thermostat in order to thrive and when metabolism slows down, weight loss slows down. But metabolism doesn't slow down in a matter of hours just because we didn't have time for breakfast or forgot to have lunch. As discussed, body cells call on glycogen stores to provide energy to keep us going. It is only when we provide the body cells with inadequate food for days on end that potential *famine* is perceived and the body goes into *preservation mode*.

The calorie cycling argument is based upon the principle that we can reduce our calorie intake for a few days prompting the body to force fat cells to release stored energy and shrink as long as we regularly *up* the calories on the fourth or fifth day to ensure the body doesn't see *famine* looming. Consequently, metabolism doesn't slow down to compensate. However, there are a couple of reasons why this method has become a bit of a *hot potato*. Firstly, there are a number of diet books and websites that imply that this is a guaranteed route to weight loss and suggest that there is no need to increase exercise levels. Some even go as far as to say that you can eat whatever you like as long as you eat very little for a few days and have all your treats on the fourth day before returning to mouse portions. This is NOT what successful, natural bodybuilders recommend. Secondly, the research that may in time prove that this theory could result in sustained fat loss would be extremely expensive to initiate and difficult to record so, until studies are funded we are pretty much in the dark. It does make some metabolic sense however and as long as top class nutritionally-rich foods form the basis of an eating plan and exercise plays a significant role, it may prove to be a significant fat loss strategy. Keep an eye on this one.

Fermentable Carbohydrates

When eaten, most carbohydrates are gradually broken down into smaller and smaller glucose molecules by digestive enzymes in the mouth, the stomach and the small intestine before being absorbed into the bloodstream, then it's off to the liver where they are either stored for later use or ferried off to body cells to create energy. Some carbohydrates however, resist much of the breakdown process, are not absorbed through the gut wall and just carry on down to the colon. These non-digestible carbohydrates (also known as fermentable carbohydrates or resistant starch) are used for fuel by the healthy bacteria in the colon in a fermentation process that produces short chain fatty acids (SCFAs) which have been shown to have a number of health benefits:-

- They are protective of colon cells and associated with less genetic damage which can lead to cancer.
- They increase mineral absorption, particularly calcium and magnesium which are important for heart and bone health.
- By feeding the healthy bacteria, growth of unhealthy bacteria and their toxic by-products is suppressed.

And importantly, from a fat loss point of view:-

- They help to slow down the pace at which digestible carbohydrates get broken down thereby reducing the counter-productive blood sugar highs and lows previously discussed.
- They increase satiety - keep us feeling fuller for longer.
- They promote bowel regularity - constipation is no friend where fat loss is desired.
- Resistant starch in a meal is associated with less fat storage after a meal.

They are big news and processed resistant starches are increasingly being used as a substitute for starch and fats in many foods on supermarket shelves. After extensive study of the available research, one American reviewer concluded that "the positive results seen in applications testing suggest that a granular resistant starch can serve many purposes in the development of healthy foods. First, as an ingredient, resistant starch provides crispness to foods such as crackers, waffles, and French toast and its expansion ability can be used to impart unique textural properties to cereals and snacks. Because of its lower caloric content, resistant starch can also be used to complement reduced-fat and reduced-sugar formulations. Second, as a functional fibre, resistant starch's white colour, fine particle size, and bland flavour make it possible to formulate food products that have more appeal and greater palatability than those made solely with traditional fibres. In this respect, resistant starch not only fibre-fortifies but imparts special characteristics not otherwise attainable in high-fibre foods. In physiological tests, resistant starch has been shown to increase fecal bulk and the production of SCFAs, such as butyrate, which is known to promote good colonic health. Finally, because of these potential physiological benefits, resistant starch may have capacity to serve as a nutritional ingredient in the development of foods that are appetizing as well as "good-for-you."

The above and other findings can only be good news for global waistlines.

Obesity is now a global issue so new ways of tackling it are going to continue to be investigated and new discoveries made that could benefit all.

Part 2. Chapter Ten

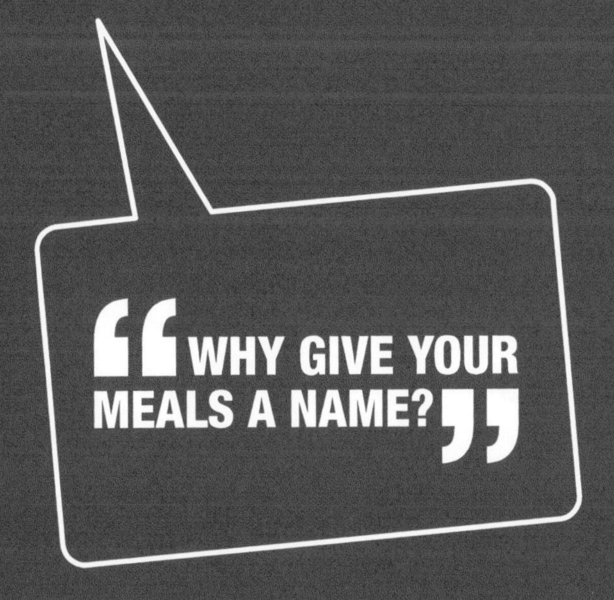

You don't have to force the porridge down at 7.30am just
because some deem it to be the perfect breakfast option!

Why Give Your Meals a Name?

Why dieting makes you fat, why prescriptive weight loss programmes are doomed to failure, why yo-yo diets and cravings for sugary, salty and fatty foods go hand in hand have all been covered. And, in the final section of the book the reasons why physical activity is a vital ingredient if you seriously want to fat burn are explained - thankfully, this does not have to involve endless hours of pounding the streets or continually turning up the speed and incline buttons on the treadmill.

Breakfast at breakfast time – why?

In this chapter we discuss how invaluable it can be to eat what you want, when you want. This probably seems at first sight a rebellious and revolutionary route to beating the bulge and you are probably thinking it cannot possibly work, but it can. Today's world would be a sad, sorry and uninteresting place if rebellion and revolution hadn't played a big part in our history. The most important thing to grasp here is that many of us have been conditioned into accepting what and when we should eat. Breakfast at breakfast time, lunch at lunchtime, dinner at dinner time and maybe a couple of light snacks mid-morning and mid-afternoon to keep body and soul together and keep hunger at bay. Various *experts* giving advice in newspapers, magazines, websites, TV and radio programmes are passionate about helping us make the right decisions when making food choices at these particular times of the day but many of the suggestions are simply low fat, low salt, low sugar versions of the US or UK breakfast, lunch and dinner classics. It doesn't have to be like that.

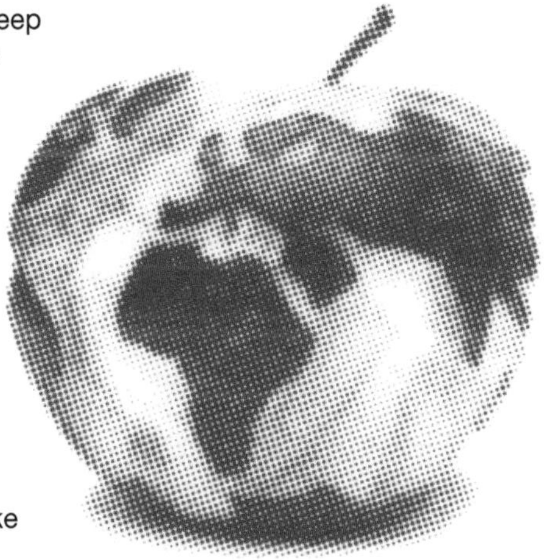

Once you understand what foods, drinks and combinations of the same work for you and boost not only your fat burning potential but also your health defences, you will be in charge - for life. No longer will you have to force the porridge down at 7.30am because some deem it to be the perfect breakfast option that will keep you fuelled all morning and fat burning until lunchtime. If you are a Scot like me, you are likely to sing the praises of porridge and recommend its consumption at **any** time of the day, but more of that and loads of ways to get fabulous fat burning oats into your diet later!

Get Global

Let's look at what our global neighbours eat for breakfast, lunch and dinner, starting with early morning. If you are in Egypt, you might well have the traditional breakfast of *Ful Mesdames*, slow cooked broad beans and lentils dressed with olive oil, lemon juice and garlic and served with a fried egg and pita bread. In Japan, most breakfasts include a bowl of steamed white rice, a small piece of salmon or other fish, a bowl of miso soup with tofu, vegetables and sometimes tiny pickled plums plus green tea. A regular Turkish breakfast includes white cheese, tomatoes, black olives, bread with honey or preserves, cured meats and an egg - all accompanied by sweet black tea. The French are devoted to their freshly baked baguettes, croissants, *pain au chocolat*, brioche or toast with creamy butter and home made preserves washed down with steaming bowls of *café au lait* or hot chocolate and in Italy, breakfast is just not a big deal. They are big on coffee in the morning, espresso or cappuccino sometimes accompanied by a pastry or a sweet biscuit.

Moving on to lunch and dinner, the choices across the globe are as vast as the foods available, dependent on where you are and the depth of your pocket but there are generally staples which form the basis of many countries' meals where there is a dependence and respect for locally grown, seasonal produce; a practice which is sadly losing its appeal in many more developed countries where junk, fast and processed foods are taking a front seat.

Having a global perspective on our food choices offers a wealth of benefits.

Lunch is the largest meal of the day in Morocco and is usually composed of *Mezze* to start - a selection of appetisers which include pita bread, hummus, olives, cheese and pistachios. *Kibbeh*, the national dish of ground lamb, spices and cracked wheat is frequently the main course but kebabs (cubes of cooked meat on a skewer) and *kefta* (ground meat mixed with herbs and spices) are popular too. *Baklava* (flaky pastry, nuts, dried fruit and honey or rose water) or a bowl of fresh melon will likely end the meal. In Sweden you will generally be offered a *smorgasbord* beginning with herring and other smoked fish followed by cold meats, salads and egg dishes. Next are hot dishes such as Swedish meatballs and cooked vegetables and lastly fruit salad or cheesecake. Goat, chicken or lamb will be on offer in Tanzania if you can afford it but the staples are rice and bean dishes with lots of greens on the side (often prepared with coconut and peanuts or tomatoes and peanut butter). Fresh fruit is usually eaten for dessert and sometimes honey or potato cakes. Most meals in Vietnam include a light broth with meat or poultry and noodles, a stir-fry or other main dish with meat, white rice and a selection of seasonal vegetables. Fresh salads abound and fresh coconut milk is often the drink of choice.

Not all the above tick the *fat busting* potential boxes but a whole lot of them do and if we adopt a global perspective to our food choices – and let's face it, it's all there on the supermarket shelves – we can *pik'n'mix* our meals and food choices according to how we feel, what we have planned, how busy we are, where we are geographically and most importantly what we feel like eating at **any time of the day, every day**.

We have discussed the *fat-gaining* potential of certain food combinations and the dangers of over-consumption of the 3 S's. These seriously are the demons when you want to lose fat from your belly, your thighs or wherever but with such a fabulous selection of alternatives they don't deserve a seat at the table.

Having your Cake and Eating it

Not possible you may say – on the contrary! Having a global perspective on our food choices offers a wealth of benefits. Every country and every culture has its strengths and weaknesses. If we take the good from some we can assemble a diet that may allow us to live longer and healthier lives. The Moroccans have one fifth the number of heart attacks we have in the UK, twice the number of Chinese die from cancer compared to India, half the number of Germans die from strokes as the Swedish and there are three times as many men, women and children classified as obese in the US as there are in Italy. Why? What can we learn from them? Of course it is not all about diet; genetics, geography, exercise levels and environmental conditions have a huge influence but eating habits play a big part.

Many of us are in the enviable position of being able to cherry-pick from the health-giving foods and recipes that form the staples in many countries where low cancer, heart attack, stroke and obesity rates exist to ensure that our diet provides the lot. Fruits and vegetables, oily fish, soy products, pulses, beans and lentils, nuts, olive oil and red wine are some of the best-researched but there are loads more which offer protection, promote fat loss and provide a diet that is so varied that boredom will never be an issue – variety is the spice of life after all!

Part 2. Chapter Eleven

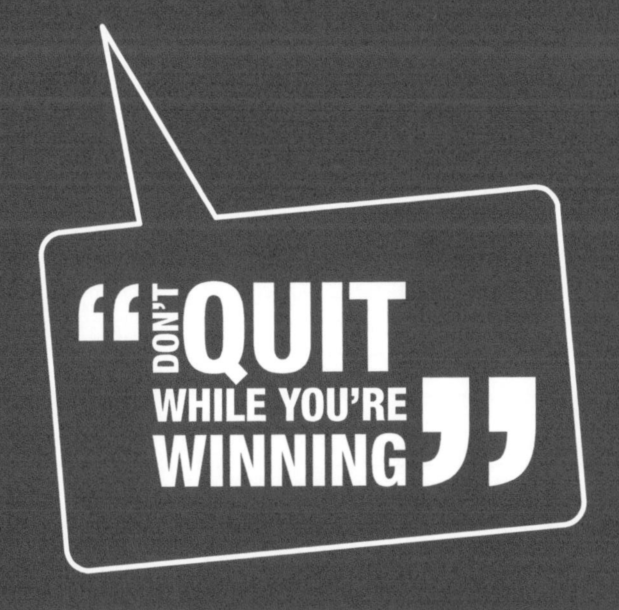

A 1000 calories of popcorn is easy, a thousand calories of cheese is a struggle!

Oh the Plateau! Disaster Strikes!

Many people trying to lose weight will hit a plateau at some stage. Why?

Imagine this scene. You are stranded on a desert island and have no food, but enough water to survive and you weigh 120lbs on day one. Let's say walking a couple of miles around the island each day to find food uses around 120kcals of energy. If you only find meagre rations you will certainly lose weight, perhaps 10lbs in the first week. So you now weigh 100lbs. Walking the same distance daily now uses less calories because you are carrying less body weight - let's say 100kcals of energy for arguments sake. Rations are still meagre and the following week you lose another 10lbs down to 90lbs and walking the same distance will probably only use up around 90kcals. What is happening in this imagined situation is that your body is continually turning down the rate at which you create energy in order to keep you alive, so when you are finally rescued four weeks later you will not have lost another 40lbs because you will have hit a plateau to preserve you.

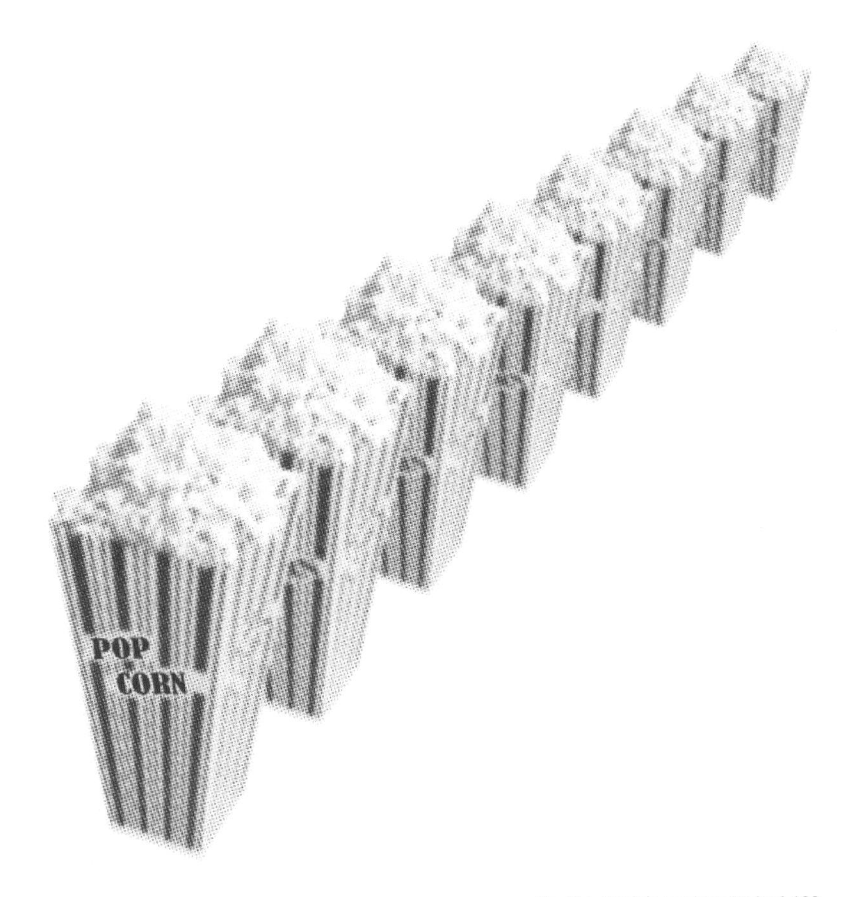

It should perhaps be called *preserving* rather than *plateauing* because that's what your body is doing. It simply cannot allow you to get into debt nutritionally otherwise you would be dead long before the rescue boat hits the shore.

This is precisely what happens when we launch into diets which repeatedly restrict calories and no matter how many lengths we swim per week or how many hours we spend on the treadmill, the plateau is just around the corner. The body responds to gradual calorie *reduction* positively but puts up a huge fight where calorie *restriction* is ongoing.

The speed with which a plateau occurs and the length of time it lasts depends on a great many factors. Age, gender, how long a person has been overweight, how long they have been on a calorie-restricted diet and how often they have yo-yo dieted are believed to be some of the main considerations. Plateauing is a period of adaptation - the body is coping with the stress of continued weight loss and adapting to the rate of energy intake in relation to energy expenditure so you have to shake it up a little.

Changing The Goalposts

Change is believed to be the best weapon here as the routine of eating, drinking and exercising in the same way daily is likely to be keeping the metabolism firing at the same pace, so no further weight is lost.

There are lots of things you can do to help you break through a plateau, here are a few that may encourage you to keep going:-

Change Your Energy Intake

- Try some totally new foods and 'google' adventurous ways to cook them.
- Change your eating patterns - have lunch at breakfast time and breakfast at lunch time etc.
- Try different drinks - experiment with smoothies and try some different teas.
- Alter your carbohydrate/protein/fat combinations for a while - less carbohydrate foods at breakfast, more protein at lunch etc.
- Change your eating haunts - go Thai, Japanese or Korean instead of Italian or American.

Change your Energy Expenditure

- Change the time of day you exercise.
- Add more weights, change the number of repetitions etc.
- Increase speed and shorten your route when out walking/jogging.
- Walk a different route to work, the shops etc.
- Walk backwards for half your exercise session.
- Stand on one leg for as long as you can when you are watching TV then swop legs.

Change Your Lifestyle

- Go to bed earlier than usual.
- Get up earlier than usual.
- Take up a new hobby, join a dance class, join a cycling club etc.
- Go on the type of holiday that you may never have even considered.

Get out of your comfort zone and enjoy the experience!

The Fat Loss Plan is designed in such a way that if you get into a bit of a routine, changes to your diet can easily be made and remember there is no such thing as one eating pattern for all. Your eating pattern is the one that fits into your life and meets your energy requirements.

Hunger + Satiety (feeling full)

Bingeing on foods that are high in protein and fat is hard. Most people can't do it. When we are faced with a plate piled high with large, fat, juicy steaks we may manage one, maybe two, possibly even three but generally we feel stuffed fairly quickly. Sadly, the same doesn't apply when it comes to starchy and sugary carbohydrates. We can eat chips, crisps, popcorn, biscuits, cakes and hot buttered toast until the cows come home and still manage just one more helping! Why is this? Why does the appetite switch that tells us we can't eat any more steaks not tell us that we can't cram in another slice of pizza?

One well-reported overfeeding experiment saw a group of people eating a whopping 10,000kcals per day of predominantly starchy, sugary carbohydrate foods and yet they were still hungry later in the day, whereas the other group who were faced with “plates of pork chops a mile high” couldn’t consume anywhere near the same number of calories. Researchers discovered that both the anticipation of the starchy, sugary foods and the actual eating of them caused the secretion of the hormone, insulin in the first group. Not only in larger amounts than the other group but more regularly. Interestingly, other experiments show that many people who are seriously overweight or clinically obese are more likely to choose sugary, starchy foods when hunger strikes.

In essence, a thousand calories of popcorn is easy, a thousand calories of cheese is a struggle.

Where the confusion lies for many trying to lose weight is that much of the advice we are bombarded with involves overly-complicated explanations of why repeated secretion of insulin into the bloodstream, to keep levels of glucose within safe limits, leads to fat storage. If you have the kind of brain that can digest the science and understand the principles of hyperinsulinism, lipogenesis, lypolysis and a host of other complex terms it may all become crystal clear and you can adopt a strategy that is going to bust the fat for good, but in my experience, many dieters are completely lost before they have reached the second page! So, let’s keep it simple.

Starchy, sugary carbohydrates satisfy our need for glucose to create energy fast when we are hungry, stressed, overtired etc. but they come at a price. They don’t sustain us for long and they don’t supply us with the level of micronutrients required to feed our energy-demanding body cells. Hunger strikes all too quickly and the brain tells us to eat. When we reach for more of the same, the process starts all over again. The pancreas continues to produce insulin to ferry the glucose out of the bloodstream and into body cells, but it gets over-worked and can’t secrete the insulin at the required pace and to make matters worse, the body cells begin to get tired of continually being asked to *unlock the gates* to receive the glucose and become less willing. So what happens next? The glucose remains in the bloodstream for too long, warning signals are sent out and the glucose is dumped wherever there is a taker. Insulin does not have to be present in order for brain cells to take in glucose so they are an easy target, but whilst they are glucose-greedy, they can have too much of a good thing and an overload can be toxic and potentially dangerous. Research into the effects of too much glucose in brain cells and its effect on our mental health continues to be well-funded as the detrimental effects becomes increasingly apparent.

From a fat loss point of view it is not good news either. When the pancreas is worn out and body cells that need to create energy are struggling to respond to the insulin instruction to take in more glucose, much of the excess is dumped in fat cells and stored.

If you want to burn fat for energy in a bid to get the fat cells to shrink you have to not only ensure that the pancreas is in good working order but also that the body cells regularly *unlock the gates*. So, how do we achieve this preferred scenario? By responding to hunger with foods that not only provide nourishment but also keep us feeling fuller for longer, don't overwork the pancreas and don't undermine the insulin response from the body cells.

We have to feed the body cells, not deprive them or confuse them.

How?

- **Give them fuel** - with energy-dense carbohydrates.
- **Eat protein with every meal and snack** - to slow down the release of glucose from the carbohydrates into the bloodstream and moderate the secretion of insulin.
- **Add essential fats** - to make us feel fuller for longer, keep hunger at bay and further moderate the insulin release.
- **Enrich them** - with foods packed with vitamins and minerals to feed the enzymes that play such an important role in efficient energy production.

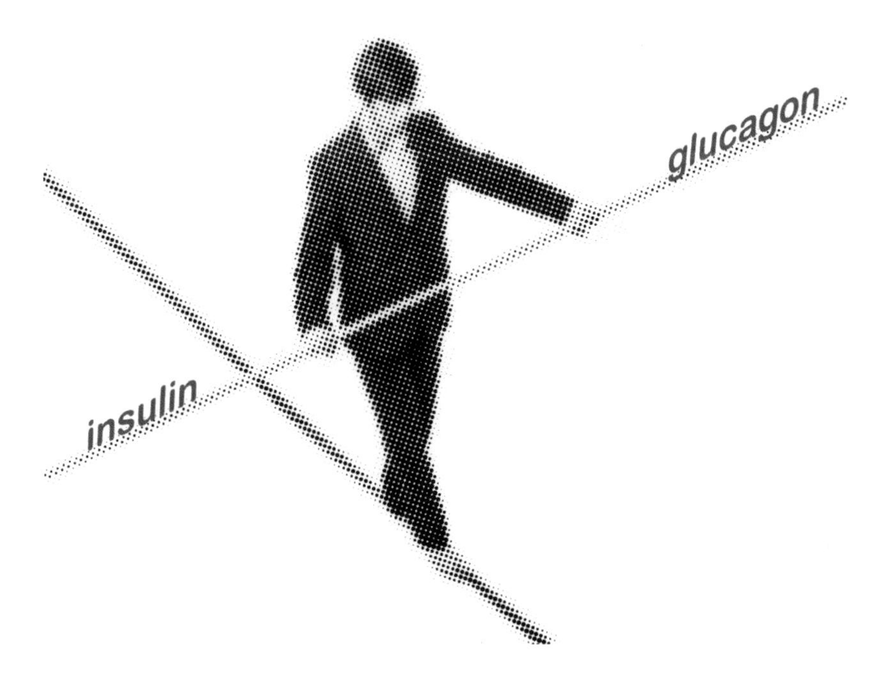

As mentioned, it is not just the continued eating of starchy, sugary carbohydrates that makes demands on the pancreas to secrete insulin, it's also the anticipation of these foods that can lead to low levels of sugar in the bloodstream and create the very real need for balance with yet more sugar. This can be dangerous for dieters, particularly when they are following low or very low calorie programmes or cutting back on certain food groups. The importance of getting a good balance of the 'Big 6' at regular intervals throughout the day can't be over-emphasised here. Keeping emergency snacks about you to counteract blood sugar lows works for most - just a piece of fruit and a handful of nuts, a cold boiled egg or a cooked chicken leg can quickly put the brakes on. See chapter 17, *What's in the Fridge etc*. and be sure to have a few of the suggestions to hand so the hunger monster doesn't take centre stage.

Cravings

The craving for starchy, sugary carbohydrates is essentially a physiological one. We see them, smell them, think about them or gorge on them and the complex network of hormones and neurotransmitters that respond to our level of hunger or satiety, our desires, our level of stress, our metabolic rate and a host of other perceived needs leaps into action. These needs often prompt a rise in blood glucose levels which have to be monitored and the pancreas is called upon to release insulin into the bloodstream to bring the level back within safe limits. While the biochemistry behind our craving for these foods is intricate and as yet unproven, many studies suggest that regularly elevated insulin levels and over-stimulation of what is often called the *reward centre* in the brain, which sees us looking for more of the same, are linked and if we don't satisfy the *need*, feelings of depression and anxiety quickly manifest themselves. This has led researchers to investigate the possible biochemical similarities between drug addiction and food addiction, which may prove invaluable in determining how cravings can be managed, in time. In the meantime, all we know for sure is that any diet that fails to control both cravings and hunger is sure to fail in the long term. Cutting back on starchy, sugary foods, concentrating on energy-dense carbohydrates and ensuring that we eat a little protein and/or essential fat with every meal and snack regulates insulin levels and by making us feel fuller and more nutritionally satisfied for longer, reduces the risks. Sticking with this practice has, over time seen an end to cravings for many and for some, even the loss of their sweet tooth!

Part 2. Chapter Twelve

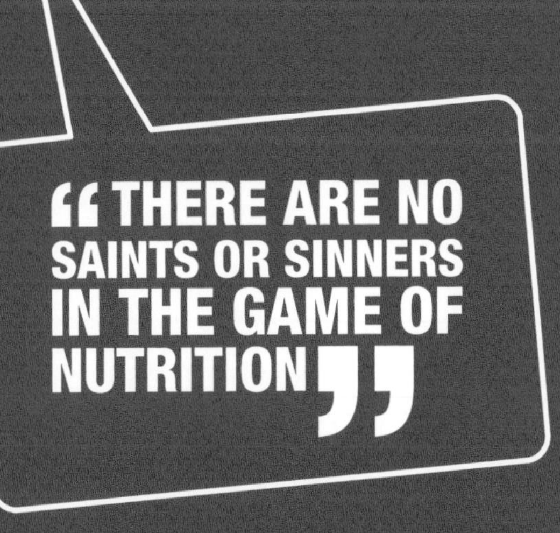

A third of Tesco shoppers dutifully eat something they cannot stomach at least once a week, believing it improves their health!

The Apple v The Cheesecake

Which is better for us and gets gold stars for nutritional value, the apple or the cheesecake? Easy - the apple. But does that make the cheesecake the bad guy? Certainly not. There's little doubt that certain slices of cheesecake don't tick many nutritional boxes and are heaving with ingredients that we can barely spell never mind recognise. But then there is the cheesecake from the local deli which has been prepared locally and lovingly using fabulously fresh eggs, cheese and cream and topped with berries that have that special scent that you know means they were picked only days ago.

That cheesecake should never be regarded as a sin.

The apple doesn't need analysis because it came straight from the tree and hasn't been processed in any way so we don't have to debate its nutritional qualities. This is where it can all get very confusing when it comes to fat loss. If a food is in anything other than its natural state, it's very hard to know what kind of processes it has been through. Some retain their health-giving properties and others can be screwed up big time. This is where reading labels is imperative.

Of course, there **are** some real saints and these are the fruits and vegetables that crowd the supermarket shelves, can be grown on the windowsill, demand 80% of the stalls at local Farmers' Markets, are grown in allotments across the UK and have definitely got the *X factor* nutritionally.

But, has the '5 a Day' marketing worked? Have you increased the number of fruits and vegetables you get into your diet on a daily basis or is your day just too damned short or busy to fit them all in?

Some polls and surveys suggest we're doing ok, others say we just haven't got to grips with it. Awareness of the 'eat more fruits and vegetables' message has exceeded expectation apparently but compliance is more than disappointing. The daily average in the UK wobbles somewhere around 2.7 portions for women, 2.5 portions for men and a mere ONE A DAY for teenagers! It's all doom and gloom from a health point of view. Another study reports that fewer than 1 in every 100 Britons meets the WHO (World Health Organisation) criteria for recommended levels not only of fruits and vegetables, which need to be increased but also saturated fats, salt and sugar which need to be reduced. Doesn't make great reading. Conversely, research commissioned by the National Consumer Council finds that two thirds of Britons have changed their eating habits or increased their exercise levels in a bid to become healthier which suggests that the spate of publicity on the health risks of obesity must be having some effect. And interestingly, a poll of over 1000 Tesco shoppers reveals that a third "dutifully eat something they cannot stomach at least once a week, believing it improves their health". Spinach, oily fish, brown bread, broccoli, Brussels sprouts, lentils, muesli, liver, mushrooms and onions top the list.

But let's look on the bright side. The media is full of encouraging stories about the increase in the number of Farmers' Markets which offer seasonal fruit and vegetables straight from 'grower to home', demand for allotments is on the rise, Hugh Fearnley Whittingstall's 'land share project' has been a fantastic success, enabling local communities to grow and enjoy their own produce and Jamie Oliver has done more than any celebrity chef to expose those who are responsible for encouraging our poor eating habits while championing affordable and workable ways to get fresh, nutritious foods into our daily diet. The 'Dinner Lady of the Year' 2009 ('Dinner Man' in this case) encouraged an 800% increase in the number of children taking his school lunches, got the kids involved and excited about growing their own vegetables and herbs on site and even introduced homemade game pie from local sustainable sources onto the menu. Britain's Best Dish 2009 was won by a 16 year old whose passion for food was infectious and one of the top selling student cookbooks was written by a teenager who certainly *knows his onions* when it comes to eating well on a budget. And hordes of students are following his lead.

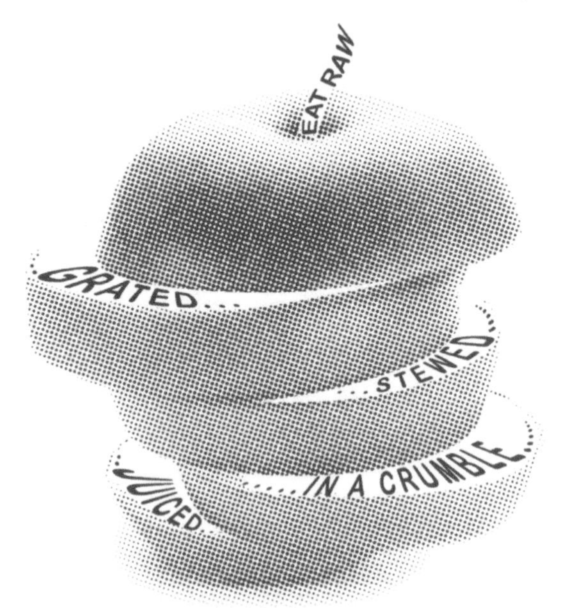

Why are fruits and vegetables so hateful?

Why was the number "5" selected as the UK goal when the Australian government recommends 7, Greece 9 and in the US, The National Cancer Institute says the minimum should be 5 for children, 7 for women and 9 for men? The French have gone one better and recommend 10! It appears to be something to do with us being such poor fruit and vegetables eaters that 5 was deemed achievable. Sadly, even 5 seems to be a step too far. So why are they so hateful, why do we resist them? They come in every colour of the rainbow and if we removed them from the supermarket shelves it would be a bleak place. Many of them can be enjoyed raw or cooked, they are as easily transported as a packet of crisps and the variety of dishes you can concoct with them is almost limitless. Susannah Blake wrote a book, published in 2008 called *5 A Day Meal Planner. More than Half a Million Delicious Recipe Combinations to ensure You and your Family get all the Fruit and Vegetables you Need* - bit of a wordy title admittedly but surely out of over half a million suggestions we can all find something that works!

Would it help if we were reminded that fruits and vegetables provide fibre, minerals, vitamins, trace elements, carotenoids, coumarins, flavonoids, indoles, lignans, isoflavones and phytosterols and that they can help prevent health problems such as depression, heart disease and cancer? Thought not! How about the fact that the wealth of coenzymes they contain are vital when it comes to breaking down the food we eat into its component parts to create energy in every cell in the body, or that their incredible antioxidant properties can help to build a strong fortress against the now well-publicised *free radicals* that threaten to invade body cells thanks to the chemicals, preservatives and twisted fats that form the basis of many of the foods people eat on the run? Possibly rather too much information to take in.

So, let's just look at their role in fat loss:-

- They achieve all of the above
- They add colour to our life and our diet
- They fill us up if we get the timing right
- They accelerate fat burning
- They reduce bloating and water retention

It appears that getting "5" into a day is a struggle, but actually getting "9" portions into a day really can be achieved without too much stress. As long as you have them in the fridge, the freezer, the handbag or briefcase, the desk drawer, the glove compartment etc. and find an opportunity to buy a couple during the working day you may be surprised when you take the time to record your consumption just how easy it was. Don't obsess about what "constitutes a portion", just go for variety and colour.

Take the versatility of apples as an example - difficult to hate, easy to love. They can be eaten whole, drunk as fresh apple juice, added to smoothies, stewed and served with yoghurt, grated over salads, stuffed with raisins and sultanas and baked in the oven, made into a crumble, put into a punch or spiced tea, added to soups, stuffings or curries, grated and added to minced pork to make burgers or meatballs, freshly sliced with cheese and fresh nuts, made into sorbets, used in chutneys, grated into coleslaw, dried and eaten as a quick snack – the list goes on.

And, how about peas? Surely everybody loves peas, fresh or frozen? They can be eaten straight from the pod, added to risottos or curries, mixed with mash, braised with leeks and other greens, incorporated into Chinese dishes, added to smoothies (that really works!) and all kinds of soups, served with rice and chicken, used to give an omelette or frittata a bit of colour, slung onto a pizza, great in a paella, smashed and spread on bruschetta with fresh tomato and cheese, mixed into noodles or pasta dishes or turned into mushy peas. And that's just for starters!

The point is that fruits and vegetables are the most versatile, nutritious and available foods on the planet and allowing them to take centre stage in our diet doesn't mean we have to crunch our way through endless raw chunks from morning until night. There are not quite 'over half a million ways' to include them in your day in chapter 14, *Lots of 'Eats'*, but there are certainly lots of tricks and tips that make sure adding them to your life isn't a chore.

Part 3. Chapter Thirteen

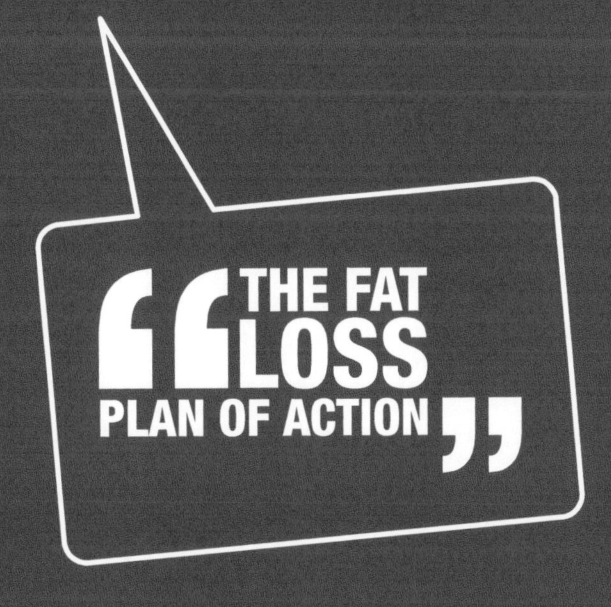

A plan that works is a plan that suits you, that you believe is going to work and that fits comfortably into your life.

Losing fat for good is not about starving or beating yourself up when you have the occasional treat and should never be about deprivation, frustration or feeling tired, hungry or nauseous. Losing fat for good is about eating great food, eating, living and loving the foods that rev up the fat busting enzymes and working out a plan that suits **you**, that **you** believe is going to work and that fits comfortably into **your** life.

It is important to note that if you are pregnant, breastfeeding, on regular medication, have concerns about your health or are under the age of 16 you should consult your doctor or health practitioner before embarking on any new eating and/or exercise programme.

So what can you expect from *The Fat Loss Plan?*

- Healthy fat loss every week
- More energy
- Improved digestion
- Clearer skin
- Sharper brain
- Better sleep

So how does it work?

The recommended 'eats' offer a combination of the foods and drinks needed to put the foot down on the metabolic accelerator and the better the quality and variety, the more efficient the machine, so you have to get the lot:-

- **Carbohydrates** for energy
- **Protein** for building and repair
- **Essential fats** for cell health and fat burning
- **Micronutrients** for protection

Eating something every 2-3 hours provides a steady flow of nutrients to the brain and body cells as well as avoiding energy dips and cravings which often lead to an overwhelming need for sweet or salty snacks.

Grazing rather than gorging keeps us energised and satisfied all day and avoids the overstuffed/sluggish feeling that often results after a large meal. Unless we are about to launch into some sort of energy-demanding activity, too much food at one sitting only increases the potential for some of that energy to be stored in the fat cells, plus the digestive system can become overburdened and less efficient. Little and often are the buzz words here.

Avoiding starchy carbohydrates after 6pm makes sense when you are 'having a night in'. They are great energy-givers when you are on the go all day but tend to make you feel bloated and uncomfortable at bedtime if you have been sitting on the couch watching TV. Plus, the insulin surge they create prompts the glucose produced to be stored as fat rather than used for energy. This means the inclusion of whole grains and fibre-rich beans, lentils and legumes during the day but not after 6pm unless you work shifts, exercise late in the evening, have an unusual work pattern, have an energetic night ahead or need a bedtime snack (the reasons why a bedtime snack may be necessary for some are covered later in this chapter).

NB: *If you are eating out, buying the occasional ready meal or grabbing food to go, avoiding starchy carbohydrates after 6pm can be tricky as you can't always be sure of the exact ingredients. If you can see them avoid them but don't obsess about them, just be alert.*

Planning ahead where possible allows you to be in charge which means you are rarely stuck in that place where the only option is fast food or a take-away on the way home.

Eating until you are only 80% full takes a bit of time to get to grips with but means less calories per day. A major study reveals that the people of Okinawa, an island off mainland Japan enjoy not only what may be the world's longest life expectancy but also the world's best health expectancy. There are more centenarians on Okinawa than anywhere else in the world and their average BMI (body mass index) is 20 - lean is less than 23. Most of them have been lean throughout their lives and one of the major influences is believed to be how much they eat. They practice a habit known as *hara hachi bu* (eating until they are only 80% full) which results in them eating around 1800kcals per day which is around 700kcals less than the average in the western world.

Using the *Waistband Method* and binning the scales removes doubt about progress. Muscle is denser than fat so as you get fitter and leaner your weight may fluctuate. The daily practice of putting on a skirt, pair of trousers or jeans with a tight waistband is a great way of measuring progress. As the weeks go by and the waistband becomes comfortable, the process can be repeated with a size smaller. This method is a great deal more satisfying than watching a little needle waver frustratingly from right to left. It only takes a few minutes and a shrinking waistline is a great way to get the day off to a good start. Even when desired fat loss has been achieved, this discipline can keep you on track.

When you make *good choices* most of the time and start losing stored fat you learn to look far beyond the calorie counting message – it's about eating great food, not about mathematics.

When you know that treats are not off limits you don't feel deprived and miserable - foodie treats should play a role in everyone's life, but perhaps not every day if you want to shift fat!

Adding warming herbs and spices to food can turn up body heat and may encourage more efficient fat burning. Making sure there are always a couple of chillies in the vegetable basket is just the start – more suggestions on how to add foods that may, in time prove to have thermogenic properties are in the next chapter, *Lots of 'Eats'*.

Regular exercise is the best-researched fat burner of them all. It's another piece of the thermogenic/fat burning jigsaw and the health-giving advantages are not in doubt, but it requires 30 minutes of your undivided attention per day. 30 minutes! Is that really too much to ask when most of us are on the go for 16 hours a day? How to get the best results from your 30 minutes is covered in chapter 15, *Your Body is Made of Moving Parts, so Move Them*.

So is it easy to follow? . . .Yes!

The Fat Loss Plan is all about thinking *outside the box* and apart from the importance of avoiding starchy carbohydrates after 6pm whenever possible offers the freedom to tailor all meals and snacks to your lifestyle – you can *pik'n'mix* as you please. Creating your own eating pattern means you don't have to stick to a rigid regime.

So what will you eat?

- **Carbohydrates for Energy** -Fruits, Vegetables, Rice and Grains, Beans, Lentils and Legumes.
- **Proteins for Building and Repair** - Fish and Shellfish, Lean Meats and Poultry, Eggs, Nuts and Seeds, Low Fat Dairy Products, Beans, Lentils and Legumes.
- **Essential Fats for Cell Health and Fat Busting** - Oily fish, Nuts plus their Oils and Butters, Seeds plus their Oils and Butters, Olive Oil, Coconut Oil, Rapeseed Oil, Avocados.
- **Micronutrients for Protection** - Plant Foods – Vegetables, Fruits, Herbs, Rice and Grains, Beans, Lentils, Legumes and their Sprouts, Nuts and Seeds.

So when will you eat?

Small and often requires a bit of organisation if you want to shed fat, but a little forward planning can reap huge rewards and the chances of you going hungry are slim. The plan is loosely based on you getting up at 7am and going to bed around 10 or 11pm but if your day is radically different, just follow the recommendation to eat something and drink something every two to three hours.

So what will reduce your chances of fat burning?

The White Stuff

The majority of white foods are refined, sugary, fatty or salty which can upset the balance of sugar in the bloodstream, impair the transfer of nutrients into and waste out of the cells, create extra work for the digestive system and reduce the chance of releasing stored fats for energy which is the ultimate goal for effective and sustained fat loss. At most, they should form 20% of your daily diet.

When you adopt the 80:20 principle, most of the foods you eat will be colourful – green, brown, blue, red, orange, purple, yellow, black and cream. Some white foods are easily recognised (white bread, white pasta, noodles and rice, biscuits, crisps, cakes, pastries, full fat milk products etc) but many are hard to spot because they are used in the production of a wide range of foods. You have to depend on your diet detective skills here and read the label. White fruits and vegetables, nuts, low fat dairy products and dairy alternatives don't fit into the above category and should be included as they are rich in health-enhancing nutrients.

So how does it all come together?

Pick out ten, fifteen or maybe twenty combinations that appeal to you.

Most people have foods they love, foods they hate, foods they have never tried or foods they have happened upon but don't rush to repeat. Start by identifying the ones you like which provide nourishment, don't rob you of energy and are already familiar to you. Look through the vast selection of 'eats' in the next chapter, *Lots of 'Eats'* and pick out ten, fifteen or maybe twenty combinations that appeal to you. Make sure they are choices that are tempting, that fit in with your daily routine and importantly, you are confident you can pick up at your local supermarket or corner shop when you are in a rush, without creating extra stress in your day. It is vital in the early stages that you don't adopt the kind of radical overnight change to your shopping, cooking and eating pattern that is likely to lessen your resolve all too quickly.

Make gradual changes

Learning to love foods that don't normally feature on your shopping list or in your restaurant choices takes time, just as losing fat takes time, but soon these small changes become habit. Don't rush into emptying the fridge, burning the biscuit tin or filling your trolley with foods you loathe; that's the road to diet misery and is almost impossible to stick to long term, even for the most disciplined amongst us.

Small and often works for many, if not most because when we know our next snack or small meal is only a few hours away we don't fret, we don't obsess and we don't stuff ourselves when we sit down to eat. Choose, taste and savour every food decision you make. If it helps, set your mobile to remind you every three hours (7am, 10am, 1pm, 4pm, 7pm, 10pm for example) and eat something, drink something and if you can, move something when the phone buzzes. See chapter 15, *Your Body is Made of Moving Parts, So Move Them* for some quick and easy ways to add to your daily physical expenditure.

7 Days In 7 Ways

Here are 7 important points that may help you keep on track. Photocopy this page, download the points from my website or put them into your mobile phone if you need a quick reminder in the first few weeks.

- Have a pre-exercise snack first thing in the morning. If you can't fit your 30 minutes of exercise in until later in the day, ignore it.
- Have a small meal or snack before you go out the door, on the way to work or as soon as you can if you are short of time, can't face food first thing in the morning or have too many commitments.
- Make small meal and snack selections that fit in with your day throughout the day. All the suggestions in the next chapter *Lots of 'Eats'* provide a good balance of macronutrients and offer the micronutrients required to nourish you and help you to burn fat so *pik'n'mix* as you please.
- Don't forget to eat something, however small every two to three hours. Keeping yourself fuelled is the best way to avoid the blood sugar swings that prompt food choices that you may regret later in the day.
- Stay hydrated throughout the day and at night if you wake. Drink water, herb, fruit, black, green or red bush tea, fresh fruit and vegetable juices and good quality black coffee.
- Don't stick to a rigid plan. When your day goes pear-shaped your eating plan can quickly follow. Make a short list of the small meals and snacks that you know can work for you no matter where you are and keep it with you so you don't get caught out. *So What's in the Fridge, Freezer etc.* in chapter 17 is packed with suggestions.
- Make sure you have the ingredients for a night time snack in stock - you may not need them but if your day has been a bit topsy turvy the hunger monster can strike and all your good intentions can fly out the window.

Adopting a new eating pattern should be inspiring, experimental and above all, confidence-boosting. Only then can you begin to reap the rewards you seek. The beauty of *The Fat Loss Plan* lies in the fact there are no hard and fast rules, you **tailor it to the rules that are presented by your daily/weekly timetable** not to a prescriptive plan I have devised for you. I don't live your life! We all have very different priorities and tastes and it is unrealistic to expect one plan to suit all - that's why many diets don't work.

So what are the secrets to permanent fat loss?

A Quick Reminder:-

- Eat something and drink something every 2-3 hours.
- Have something to eat within 2 hours of rising.
- Check your waistband every morning.
- Recognise your hungriest times of the day and plan accordingly.
- Keep portable snacks in your handbag, briefcase, desk drawer etc.
- Eat until you are only 80% full.
- Use smaller plates and pile the plate high with vegetables and salad stuffs.
- Eat a rainbow of colourful foods and keep white foods to a minimum.
- Go for fresh, unprocessed foods whenever possible.
- Don't deprive yourself of treats but make sure they are top quality.
- Exercise for 30 minutes per day, six days a week; preferably first thing in the morning.

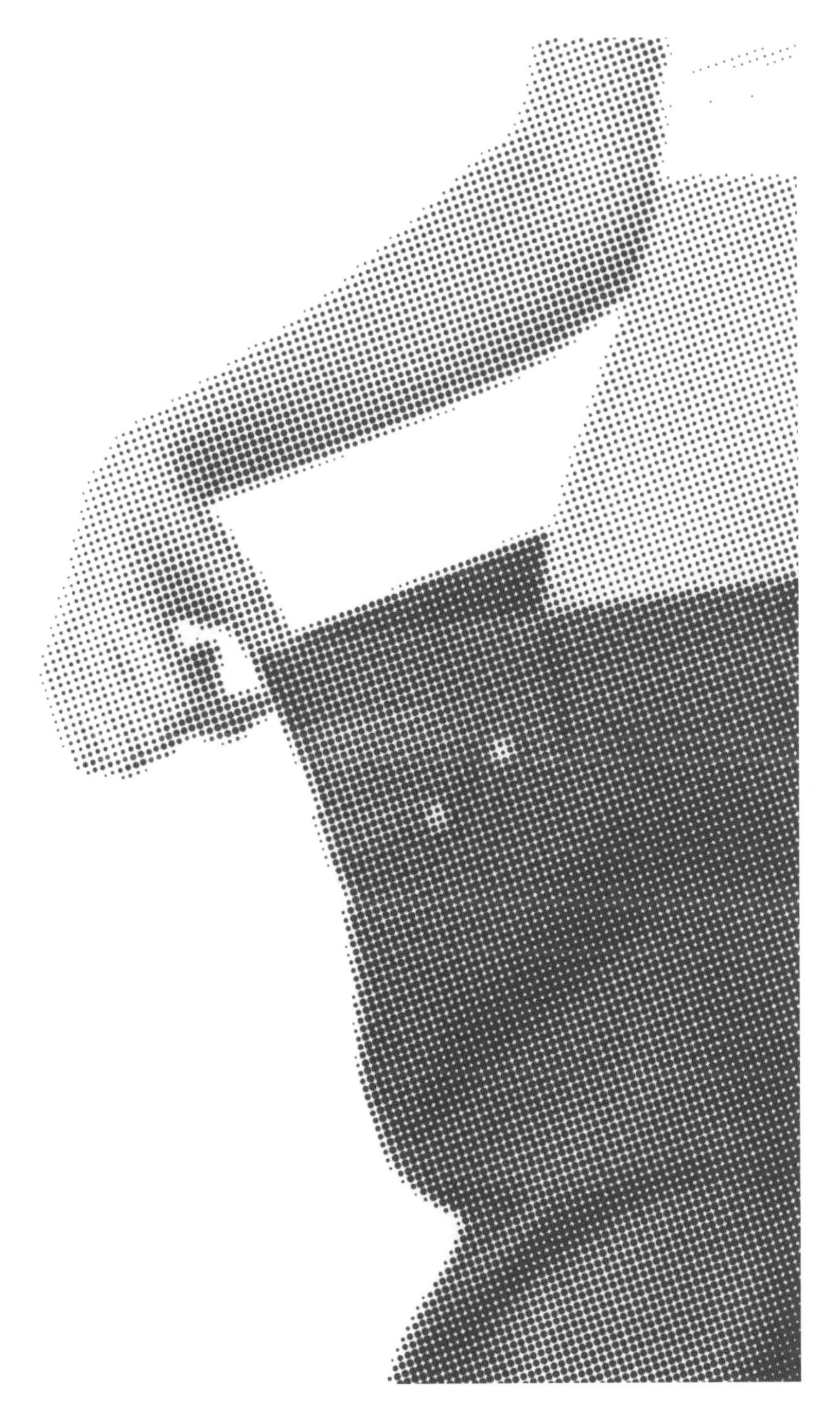

Part 3. Chapter Fourteen

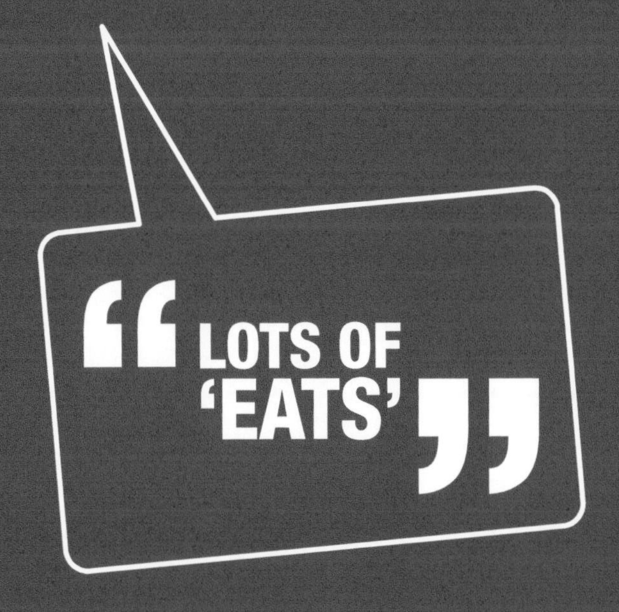

Recognising your energy dips that see you reaching for an iced doughnut like a women 'obsessed' makes good food choices a whole lot simpler.

There's no shortage of variety here and you may find the selection a bit daunting at first sight but I urge you take an experimental approach. You may find it easier to select only those that appeal from two or three sections for the first few weeks to cut down on shopping, cooking and decision-making before expanding your list and trying a few more. When you define the foods and eating practices that work for you, fit in with your lifestyle and avoid energy dips as recommended earlier in the book making these choices becomes simpler. Chapter 17, *So What's in the Fridge/Freezer etc*. is designed to ease the transition and ensure you always have foods to hand that can help you achieve your fat loss goal. Try to make a few changes every week.

Pre-Exercise 'Eats'

If you exercise first thing in the morning

- Couple of oatcakes with a slice of ham and a slice of goats cheddar.
- One sesame seed Ryvita with almond butter and sliced tomato.
- One slice of rye toast with mackerel pate and sliced cucumber.
- A piece of fresh fruit with a handful of fresh nuts.
- Small pot of natural yoghurt with a handful of berries and toasted flaked almonds.
- Small bowl of 'cold oats' (page 200).
- Sliced carrots, peppers and cucumber with a small pot of hummus.

Breakfast 'Eats'

Oat Breakfasts

Special Porridge (page 199)

Cold Oats (page 200)

Honeyed Muesli (page 201)

Porridge Smoothie (page 200)

Fruit Breakfasts

Chopped/sliced fresh fruit topped with natural yoghurt and a handful of nuts and seeds.

Dried fruit salad soaked overnight in tea and topped with low fat crème fraiche and toasted flaked almonds.

Natural cottage cheese with pineapple, mango and papaya slices.

Melon boats with parma ham slices.

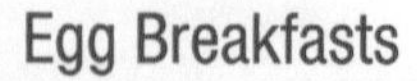

Egg Breakfasts

2 boiled, scrambled or poached eggs with rye toast and a little butter.

French toast topped with sliced peaches.

2 egg omelette with diced ham and green peas.

2 slices lean grilled bacon and scrambled egg with grilled tomatoes and mushrooms.

Liquid Breakfasts

Home made smoothie of mixed fresh fruits with a tablespoon of natural yoghurt/whey protein powder or a handful of bean sprouts added.

Essential Smoothie (page 205).

Shop bought smoothie with yoghurt and a handful of fresh nuts.

V8 or carrot juice and a couple of oatcakes with nut butter.

Cereal Breakfasts

No sugar Muesli mix with added dried fruits, nuts and seeds with chilled low fat milk or soya/rice milk.

Weetabix, Shredded Wheat, Bran Flakes or All Bran with low fat milk or nut/oat milk and a handful of fresh berries.

Millet porridge (page 199 but substitute oats with millet).

Continental + Fish Breakfasts

Pumpernickel bread toasted topped with a couple of slices of ham and a slice of hard cheese.

Small bowl of hummus with carrot sticks, fresh olives and cubes of feta cheese.

Whole wheat bagel, halved and toasted, spread with low fat cream cheese and topped with smoked salmon.

Grilled kippers.

Pickled herrings with rye toast soldiers.

'On the Go' Breakfasts

A piece of fresh fruit, a small pot of natural yoghurt and a small bag of fresh nuts and seeds.

Cold Oats (page 200) or Porridge Smoothie (page 200) in an air-tight container.

Soya milk latte and a fresh fruit salad mix.

Ready made vegetable, bean or meat soup.

Quick 'Eats'

Anytime

- Raw baby vegetables with hummus, tzatziki, natural yoghurt or salsa.
- Cold cooked chicken leg, thigh or breast (skin off) and a few baby tomatoes.
- Mini pita pocket filled with rocket, cucumber, peeled prawns and natural yoghurt.
- Mixed olives with feta cheese.
- Small pack of low salt popcorn and a handful of grapes.
- Handful of cherries with a few slices of goats cheese cheddar.
- Ryvita spread with scraping of mayo topped with tuna and sliced tomatoes.
- Rice cake with mashed banana topped with flaked almonds.
- 3 bean or rice salad from the deli.
- Low sugar baked beans on dark brown toast.
- French toast topped with peaches.
- Half an avocado stuffed with salsa and topped with crispy bacon bits (fat drained off).
- Sliced apple with a handful of mixed nuts and seeds and a chunk of hard cheese.
- Boiled egg and dark brown toast soldiers.
- Cup of *Marigold Vegetable Bouillon* with a tablespoon of miso paste.
- Tomato and basil soup with a couple of handfuls of tinned lentils.
- Bowl of home or ready made soup – see Get Soupy on page 160 for suggestions.
- Fingers of melon wrapped in parma ham.
- Quick cook couscous (tomato, roasted vegetable, Moroccan etc.) – add cooked chicken, prawns or tuna.
- Small tray of sushi – vegetable or fish.
- Tomato, basil and mozzarella salad drizzled with olive oil.

- Quick egg noodles with cubes of chicken, pine nuts, ready-roasted peppers and sun dried tomatoes and a splash of soy sauce.
- Multigrain toast with sugar free jam and a few shavings of parmesan.
- Bowl of wholegrain cereal with chilled milk topped with fruit and nuts.
- A small bowl of mixed leaf salad sprinkled with lemon juice and olive oil with a spoonful of cottage cheese and pineapple.
- Hot steaming whole wheat, buckwheat, corn or rice pasta with basil or rocket pesto.
- Small bowl of pretzels or bluecorn tortilla chips with salsa dip.
- Mixed nuts and raisins or mixed nuts and seeds.
- Top some mixed leaves with tinned mixed beans and tinned tuna and sprinkle with olive/nut oil and chilli flakes.
- Hard boil a few eggs at one time and have a cold boiled egg as a snack.
- Mix a packet of microwaveable rice with a tin of mixed beans and some spaghetti sauce, salsa or tinned tomatoes.
- Bowl of mixed berries with shelled pistachios thrown over.
- Natural cottage cheese and sliced fresh pears with sea salt and black pepper - just try it!
- Fresh dates with a couple of squares of really good dark chocolate.
- Cold Greek yoghurt with sliced bananas and toasted flaked almonds.
- Couple of oatcakes with tinned salmon and cucumber.
- Pumpernickel bread, toasted and spread with tzatziki and topped with thinly sliced smoked salmon and some cucumber or avocado slices.
- Stir a handful of raisins, some chickpeas and a few toasted pine nuts into cold cooked brown rice. Drizzle with chilli oil and throw on some chopped parsley.
- Juices and smoothies – see *Liquid 'Eats'* on page 134.

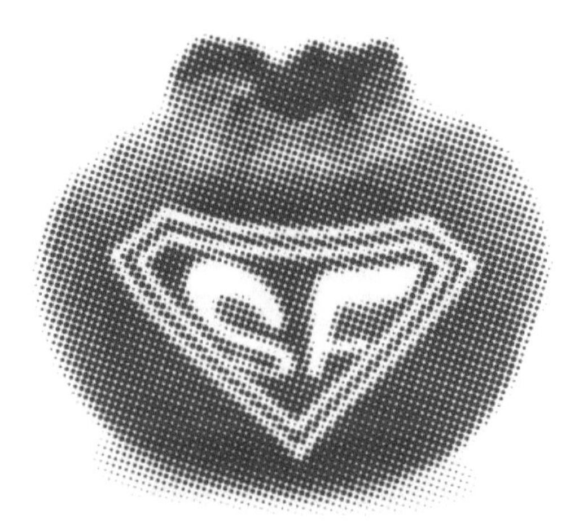

Quick 'Eats'

After 6pm (no starchy carbohydrates included)

- Raw baby vegetables with tzatziki, natural yoghurt or salsa.
- Cold cooked chicken leg, thigh or breast (skin off) and a few baby tomatoes.
- Bowl of mixed olives with feta cheese.
- Handful of cherries with slices of goats cheese.
- Half an avocado stuffed with salsa and topped with crispy bacon bits (fat drained off).
- Sliced apple with a handful of mixed nuts and seeds and a chunk of hard cheese.
- Cup of *Marigold Vegetable Bouillon* with a tablespoon of miso paste stirred in.
- Bowl of home or ready made soup – see Get Soupy on page 158 for suggestions.
- Fingers of melon wrapped in parma ham.
- Tomato, basil and mozzarella salad.
- A plate of steamed baby vegetables splashed with a few drops of balsamic vinegar and a glug of nut or seed oil.
- A small bowl of mixed leaf salad sprinkled with lemon juice and olive oil with a spoonful of cottage cheese and pineapple.
- Mixed nuts and raisins or mixed nuts and seeds.
- Hard boil a few eggs at one time and have a cold boiled egg as a snack.
- Bowl of mixed berries with shelled pistachios thrown over.
- Cottage cheese and sliced pears with sea salt and black pepper.
- Fresh dates with a couple of squares of really good dark chocolate.
- Cold Greek yoghurt with sliced bananas and toasted flaked almonds.
- Juices and smoothies – see *Liquid 'Eats'* on page 134

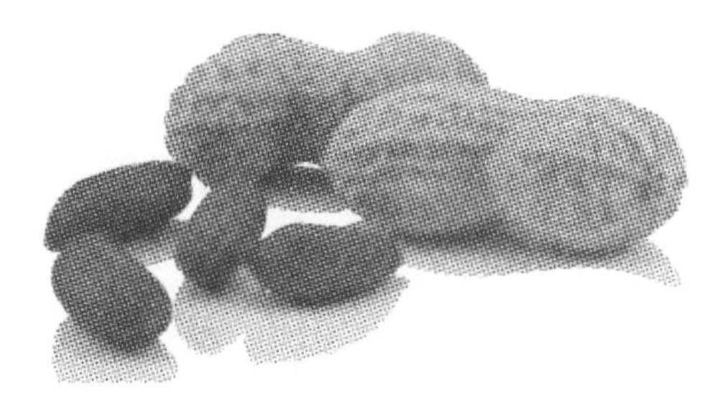

Wrapped 'Eats'

Sandwiches etc

Breads - granary, wholemeal, whole-wheat, multigrain, multi-seed, sourdough, rye, German breads, 'women's' breads, nut and seed breads. Other useful 'wrappers' - Wholemeal Pitta Pockets, Whole wheat Bagels,Tortilla Wraps.

Spread – to moisten use olive oil, crème fraiche, natural yoghurt, guacamole, salsa, hummus, tzatziki, peanut butter, nut butters and oils, pesto, cottage cheese or a scraping of butter or mayo.

Stuff – with lettuce, rocket, watercress, spinach, fresh parsley or herbs, spring onions, Chinese leaves, fennel, mustard cress, cucumber, tomatoes, grated carrot, apple or courgette, raw or grilled peppers, bean sprouts, green beans, sliced mushrooms.

Add – cooked chicken or turkey, avocado slices, tuna, cooked or smoked salmon, sardines, smoked mackerel, thinly sliced ham, prawns, grated hard cheese, mozzarella, feta, roast lean lamb or beef, hummus, chopped boiled egg or scrambled egg, crabmeat.

Sprinkle – nuts, seeds, lemon or lime juice, olive oil, sea salt, ground black pepper, chilli flakes, Tabasco, cayenne or curry powder, soy sauce, balsamic vinegar.

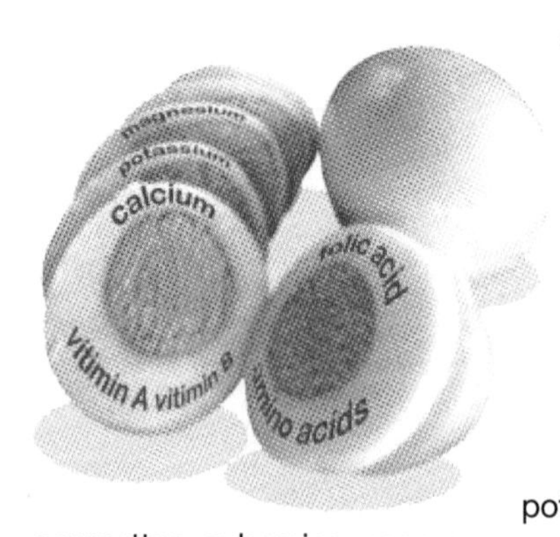

'Eats' on Stix

Buy – wooden skewers (around 10-12" long) and always soak them for about 15mins in water to stop them from burning.

Chop/Slice/Cube – pieces of chicken or chicken wings, lamb, beef, meaty fish, shellfish, prosciutto, 100% meat sausages, chicken livers, peppers, mushrooms, small part-cooked potatoes, baby onions, garlic cloves, chillies, courgettes, aubergine, asparagus, sugar snap peas, baby corn, leeks, fennel, celery, apple, pineapple, prunes, banana, tomatoes, artichoke hearts, cheese, cooked quails eggs, dense bread.

Experiment with combinations of the above, turn all the pieces in a little olive oil, thread them onto skewers and grill (15/20 mins should do it). Turn them regularly and let them rest for about 5 mins before serving on a bed of brown basmati rice.

For sweet fruity kebabs thread chunks of fruit onto the skewers, sprinkle lightly with icing sugar and grill for about 5 mins – keep an eye on them as they have a nasty habit of burning. Serve with creamy natural yoghurt.

Cold 'Eats'

There are plenty of cold 'eats' in the QUICK 'EATS' section but here are a few more. Salads are really quick, stave off pangs of hunger or can be more substantial when you need a good feed. The possible combinations are as varied as the textures and tastes.

Salads

Base – all kinds of lettuce, spinach leaves, watercress, rocket, fresh parsley and mixed herbs, sliced fennel, spring onions, sliced red onions, Chinese leaves, pak choy, mustard cress, baby gem lettuce, chicory leaves, celery leaves, chives, shredded cabbage, celery, finely sliced leeks.

Next – tomatoes (fresh and sun-dried), cucumber, bean sprouts, green beans, white beans, red beans, chick peas, lentils, new potatoes, grated carrot, grated apple, grated courgettes, radishes, red, yellow and orange peppers, sweet corn, baby corn, sugar snap peas, mangetout, mild chillies, peas, raisins, sliced oranges, sliced pineapple, sliced peaches, sliced pears, sliced mangoes, grapes, sliced avocado, baby asparagus, cold cooked pasta, noodles or rice, couscous, bulgur wheat, sliced mushrooms, artichoke hearts, olives, roasted vegetables.

Consider – cold cooked chicken or turkey, cold sliced duck or game, crisp bacon bits, lean cooked meats, hard cheeses (cubed, sliced or grated), feta cheese, goats cheese, mozzarella, cottage cheese, cooked peeled prawns, flaked fish, anchovies, sardines, fresh or tinned tuna, crab or salmon, sliced or chopped boiled egg, cubes of pancetta.

To Finish – slug of extra virgin olive oil or nut/seed oil, lemon or lime juice, balsamic, cider or fruit vinegar, sea salt flakes, ground black pepper, soy sauce, nuts (whole, toasted, chopped or flaked), seeds, dollop of mayo, crème fraiche, natural yoghurt or cottage cheese, wholegrain mustard, crushed garlic or ginger, drizzle of honey, spoonful of fruity/spicy chutney or creamed horseradish, spoonful of peanut butter, tahini, hummus or tzatziki, shake of chilli or curry powder, Worcester sauce, Tabasco, tomato puree, sprinkling of chopped herbs.

NB: If you are taking a salad to work, school or you are out and about, keep the dressing separate and add just before devouring.

Cold Oats 'n' Stuff

Some would call this a breakfast dish, but it is quite delicious and filling at any time of the day (before 6pm). You will find the method in the Recipe section.

Hot 'Eats'

Salads - use all the suggestions for cold salads but throw in some hot food for variety – chicken, prosciutto, lean lamb, chunks of minced beef, cubes of black pudding, grilled fish and shellfish (tuna, mackerel, sardines, anchovies, prawns, scallops etc), roasted peppers and other vegetables, hot new potatoes, sautéed onion slices, warm freshly boiled eggs or a perfect runny poached egg, steamed vegetables (asparagus, French beans, peas, mangetout, baby corn), hot rice or pasta, hot toasted nuts and seeds, warm beans or lentils **and/or** warm your oils (olive, nut or seed) very gently and mix through your salad at the last minute.

Soups – Some were already mentioned in the Quick 'Eats' section. You may only have time for bought soups and there is such a vast choice that you could have soup every day for a year and never have the same one twice. Watch out for the creamy, fatty, sugary, salty ones – the only way to know is to read the label or ask. Even better, make your own (recipes at the back of the book).

Omelettes and Frittatas with any or all of the following:- crumbled feta cheese, parsley, fresh herbs, rocket, cooked spinach, sautéed onions, cooked skinless chicken or turkey, grated courgettes, sliced fresh or bottled peppers, fresh or sun dried tomatoes, roasted baby vegetables, crispy grilled lean bacon or pancetta, sautéed mushrooms, steamed asparagus tips, cooked frozen peas, shavings of parmesan cheese, sliced cold cooked baby new potatoes. There is simply no-one like Delia Smith when it comes to precise instructions on making any dish you may be nervous about attempting so rather than providing recipes for omelettes and fritattas I suggest you head straight to her website. You will become an expert in no time!

Mejadarra – a lentils and rice dish with tons of flavour – see recipe section

Risottos - learn the art of making risottos and become everybody's best friend - there is no point in making risotto for one. It's a job that requires a bit of care and attention and a bottle of white wine to be shared between the dish, the chef and whoever else! There are loads of YouTube videos on how to make the perfect risotto - have a look. There are also a couple of suggestions in the recipe section which involve less butter and cheese than the 'classics'.

Stir Fries – these can be as simple or as complicated as you wish to make them. They are quick (apart from the very important preparation of everything before you start) and if you use really fresh ingredients and follow the advice of the *experts* (the Wagamama Cookbook is a great investment), they are delicious and there are very few people, including kids who can say no to a stir fry. Plus, they are a great way to get at the very least '3 a day' into just one meal.

Liquid 'Eats'

Juices, Shakes + Smoothies – the fresher the better. If you have a juicer you can extract the goodness from just about any fruit or vegetable. Alternatively, a blender will produce great results with the softer varieties of fruits and vegetables. To make them more of a meal you can add yoghurt, cottage cheese, brewer's yeast, wheat germ, molasses, tahini, non-dairy milks (soya, rice, oat, nut, coconut), lecithin powder, nut butters, spirits and more.

Seek out your nearest juice bar if time is short and experiment with some of the great combinations on offer. There are also loads of ready made juices and smoothies on the shelves but some are better than others. Generally speaking, the freshest, purest ones are the most expensive so head for them when and if you can afford them (you will often find them in the knock-down price section when their 'sell by' date is perilously close). However, a poor imitation of a fresh juice is still going to be a better choice than a can of Coca Cola!

A book is a great help when it comes to getting the combinations right. There are a couple of recommendations at the back of the book and of course, the internet is a quick and easy way to get started.

Stuffed 'Eats'

Stuff baked potatoes, sweet potatoes, tomatoes, peppers, squash, mushrooms, aubergines, courgettes or fresh bananas, peaches, dates, avocado with a variety of extras to provide a more filling meal or snack.

Potatoes + Sweet Potatoes:-

- Tinned tuna, natural yoghurt and diced cucumber.
- Lean crispy bacon and sautéed chopped mushrooms.
- Ratatouille.
- Cooked prawns, scrambled egg and black pepper.
- Strips of lean grilled beef and horseradish.
- Roasted mixed vegetables.
- Cottage cheese and herbs.
- Steamed spinach and chopped egg.
- Smoked fish and baby tomatoes.
- Diced avocado, chopped spring onions, pimientos, crumbled feta and coriander leaves.
- Cooked lentils, peas and low fat crème fraiche.

Red, Yellow, Green or Orange Peppers, Courgettes, Aubergines, Tomatoes or Squash

- Cooked brown rice, quinoa, bulgur wheat or couscous.
- Add some flaked tuna, shredded chicken, diced lean bacon, lean minced beef or lamb, lentils or beans.
- Bind with sautéed onions and garlic and top with breadcrumbs or chopped nuts.

Mushrooms

- Use large flat mushrooms and take out the stalk, chop it finely with spring onions and stir fry quickly in a teaspoon of oil.
- Mix in some shredded baby spinach and fresh breadcrumbs or chopped nuts.
- Scoop onto mushrooms, sprinkle with lemon juice and grill.
- Try adding a little minced ham, some herbs and some cheese shavings for variety.

Avocado

- Smoked fish with yoghurt and cucumber.
- A few cooked bacon bits with salsa.
- Some chopped baby tomatoes with crumbled feta.
- Hummus and diced red pepper.
- A few fresh herbs and a drizzle of balsamic vinegar.

Banana

- Cut a banana in half lengthwise (but not through the bottom layer of skin).
- Place 4 bits of darkest Green & Blacks Chocolate along the centre.
- Wrap the banana in tin foil.
- Bake in a medium oven for about 10 mins (turn it once).
- A REAL TREAT!

Peaches

- Crush a couple of amaretti biscuits.
- Mix with a teaspoon of ricotta cheese.
- Stuff the stoned peach half.
- Drizzle with honey.
- Grill for 6-7 mins.

Dates

- Stuff with pecans, almonds, pistachios or Brazil nuts and eat.

Parcelled 'Eats'

Food in Parcels (en papillote)

Cut sheets of foil or baking parchment to size (big enough to wrap the foods, seal the edges tightly and leave space for the steam to do the cooking) then lightly brush the sheets with oil.

Base - all kinds of vegetables left whole if small, chopped into cubes if accompanying meat or poultry, sliced thinly to go with fish and sliced very thinly or grated if you are using seafood.

Next – fish fillet or fish steak, sardines, scallops, 'queenies', uncooked prawns, mussels, skinless chicken, turkey or duck breast left whole or sliced into strips, lean beef, lamb, pork or organic liver sliced thinly.

Top With – fresh herbs, grated fresh ginger, lemon, lime or orange juice and zest, garlic cloves or puree, soy sauce, whole or ground spices, toasted nuts and seeds, sea salt (or alternatives), ground black pepper, thai fish sauce, dry white wine or red wine, honey, tomato puree, balsamic vinegar, green or black olives, capers, Tabasco, mustard, vegetable stock (*Marigold Vegetable Bouillion*), apple or pineapple juice, chopped dried fruits.

- Make sure you have moistened the food but don't have a pool of liquid at the bottom.
- Make sure the edges of the parcel are secure so the steam doesn't escape.
- Make sure there is plenty of space for the steam to do the cooking (it's not supposed to look like a perfectly wrapped Christmas present!)
- Lay the parcels on a baking tray and put in the centre of a preheated oven (200C/400F/gas mark 6) until cooked (have a peek inside one of the parcels to make sure!)
- 10-12 mins:- sardines, scallops, 'queenies', mussels, uncooked prawns and other shellfish.
- 15-20 mins:- fish fillets and fish steaks.
- 20 mins:- sliced chicken, turkey or duck breast, lean strips of beef, lamb, pork or organic liver.
- 25-30 mins:- whole chicken/duck breast or halved turkey breast.

Light Dinner 'Eats'

If you like a more classic 'meat and two vegetables' type of dinner, the following may appeal. But remember this is the time of the day to say no to starchy carbohydrates where possible. The combination of a decent portion of good quality protein, some essential fats and plenty of vegetables provides a filling meal that gives the body everything it needs to rest, repair and fat burn all night.

*If you are only able to fit your half hour of exercise into the early evening and usually have your meal afterwards, work shifts, have an energetic evening ahead or choose to have any of the following at lunchtime, add a cupful of brown rice, barley, couscous, beans or lentils or baked sweet potato chips (paint with olive oil and bake in a fairly hot oven until crisp round the edges and succulent inside).

- A steamed skinless turkey or chicken breast topped with pesto or olive paste.
- A poached, baked or grilled salmon fillet or salmon steak painted with Worcestershire Sauce.
- Grilled white fish fillets topped with lemon juice and a spoonful of warmed tomato salsa.
- A venison fillet or venison steak marinated for at least 10 minutes in olive oil, a couple of splashes of balsamic vinegar and ground black pepper, then grilled.
- A couple of smoked mackerel fillets baked in the oven until hot.
- Half a dozen fresh prawns coated with chilli oil and grilled.
- A 2 egg omelette or frittata with sliced courgettes, mushrooms, peppers, spinach and a few shavings of parmesan cheese.
- Tofu with garlic and ginger – cut firm tofu into cubes and stir fry in a little olive oil mixed with crushed garlic and grated fresh ginger. Add a squeeze of runny honey and top with toasted flaked almonds.
- Beef or soya mince burger – use freshly ground lean beef, minced or soya mince which has been soaked for half an hour as per packet instructions. Add some sea salt crystals, ground black pepper then other spices of choice (cumin, coriander, curry powder, chilli powder etc), plus a few shakes of Lea & Perrins or balsamic vinegar. Mould into burger shapes and chill for 20 minutes before grilling. Top with a slice of goats cheese cheddar towards the end of cooking.

Have at least 3 different steamed, grilled, stir fried or roasted vegetables (not potatoes, sweet potatoes, root vegetables or corn - too starchy unless the above applies*) and/or a large mixed salad. Top your vegetables or salad with roasted mixed nuts or seeds or mixed bean sprouts and drizzle with nut or seed oil (avocado, sesame, sunflower, pumpkin, walnut, flax, hemp etc.) and a squeeze of lemon/lime juice.

Night Time 'Eats'

Only if you are really hungry, find you can't get to sleep or regularly wake up in the wee small hours and can't get back to sleep. The following food combinations are rich in the amino acid, *tryptophan* which encourages the production of the *sleepy* chemical, *serotonin* plus if your blood sugar is all over the place can help to get the balance right overnight. Have your snack at least 30 minutes before you go to bed. You will probably find after a week or so you will be sleeping better and it won't be required:-

- A small tub of natural cottage cheese with a handful of mixed seeds.
- One egg lightly scrambled on an oatcake.
- A mug of Green & Black's hot chocolate made with soya milk (don't add sugar).
- A small carton of natural 'live' yoghurt with a swirl of honey.
- 2 or 3 squares of dark chocolate (70% cocoa solids minimum) and a few shavings of parmesan cheese.
- A small plate of porridge made with water and topped with a spoonful of *Manuka* honey.
- A couple of mini oatcakes with nut or seed butter and a couple of slices of cold turkey breast.

Tr'eats'

- Muffins, Waffles and pancakes – buy the whole grain packet mixes.
- Cereal bars (some are great, others are loaded with sugar - read the label).
- Poached fruit.
- Fresh fruit dipped in 70% dark melted chocolate.
- Berry Compotes (again watch the sugar content).
- Halved peaches filled with crushed amaretti biscuits and grilled.
- Fruit crumbles (use muesli mixes, a little butter and honey for topping).
- Plates of chopped, sliced and whole fruits with slices of cheese (ricotta, feta, parmesan) drizzled with honey.
- Dates filled with pecans, almonds or walnuts.
- French toast with poached or fresh fruit.
- Fresh cherries in a huge bowl of ice.
- Home made or good quality bought carrot cake, banana cake or fruit loaf.

Fat Busting Extras

Below is a list of foods and drinks which may boost metabolism, have thermogenic qualities or rev up fat burning enzyme activity. Some have met the exacting demands of scientific research, some are just beginning to gain ground and others have merely sparked attention but they all offer a wealth of nutrients and even if their fat busting qualities are never 100% proven, they all pack a nutritional punch. Get them into your day when you can, particularly the herbs, spices and seeds.

Apples and Pears are both high in pectin which may help reduce fat absorption and are high in soluble fibre which keeps you feeling fuller for longer.

Bananas are rich in magnesium which is essential for calcium absorption – a good balance of these two minerals is important for fat metabolism, bone and heart health.

Grapefruit, Blueberries and Tomatoes are packed with Vitamin C which may prevent fat storage and promote fat loss.

Broccoli and Celery are very rich in calcium, a possible 'big player' in fat metabolism and vitamin C which boosts calcium absorption.

Carrots are the perfect raw snack to keep hunger at bay – easy to transport, widely available, can be eaten alone or with healthy dips and their natural sweetness can help counteract cravings.

Sprouts, Cabbage, Spinach, Parsley, Beets and Cucumber are natural diuretics. Water retention can be a real problem, particularly for women, due to fluctuating hormone and fluid levels. Too much salt in the diet adds to the problem. Eating vegetables that help to keep the fluid levels balanced is important. The minerals in these vegetables may relieve bloating, improve waste management and aid fat loss.

Almonds and Walnuts have high levels of fibre, protein and essential fats – a great fat burning combination which make these nuts a great balanced and filling snack.

Flax Seeds and Sunflower Seeds contain an excellent combination of the healthy fats needed for fat metabolism but are also a great source of high quality protein and fibre.

Oats and Barley are a good source of fermentable carbohydrates and soluble fibre which research has shown to be important for fat loss.

Quinoa is not only a fibre-rich grain but is also, unusually for grains, a complete protein. Countless studies have shown that a little protein with every meal and snack may help boost metabolism, aid fat loss and build lean muscle tissue so we burn more calories.

Soybeans contain lecithin, which may prevent fat from forming in the cells and break down fatty deposits in the body.

Garlic and Garlic Oil contain a substance called allicin which research has shown to have a significant protective quality to cells helping to reduce fatty deposits.

Soup is a great appetite suppressant if you snack on it or have it as a starter. One study shows that those who chose to have soup as a snack before lunch consumed 100 fewer calories during the meal than those who made other choices.

Oily Fish is a great source of Omega 3 essential fats, now gaining ground for their fat busting qualities.

Kelp and Seaweeds feed the thyroid gland which plays an important role in efficient metabolism.

Water The rate at which we burn calories may increase when we drink water regularly throughout the day plus when are well hydrated we are less likely to be hungry.

Green Tea A few studies show that green tea extract can boost metabolism and aid fat loss.

Red Wine The seeds in grapes can have an inhibiting effect on fat gain (1 glass per day is all that's required however!)

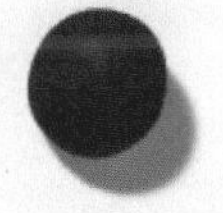

Cayenne Pepper, Paprika, Chillies, Chilli Powder and Chilli Flakes

The *capsiate* in chilli peppers has been shown to increase metabolic rate.

Cinnamon, Ginger, Black Pepper, Mustard and Horseradish

Turn up body temperature and promote good digestion. Cinnamon has also been shown to have a regulatory effect on blood sugar.

Apple Cider Vinegar

A couple of trials indicate that taking this vinegar before a meal creates a feeling of fullness so reducing the amount of food consumed. It can also aid digestion.

Part 3. Chapter Fifteen

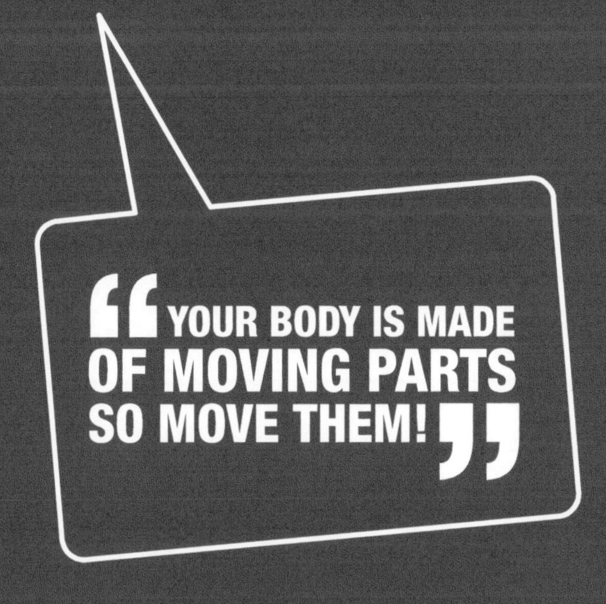

Fat cells are very happy to store energy on your hips and bum until they are called into action so if you want to wake up those fat cells, you have to gain muscle.

Fidgeting Makes You Thin!

Perhaps a bit of an exaggeration but it make some sense. Your body is moving all the time; even when you are asleep your heart is beating, your lungs are expanding and retracting, your liver works tirelessly around the clock and every movement requires energy – even the flicker of an eyelash. Where does that energy come from? Your mitochondria. These powerhouses within every living cell take in the nutrients from food and turn them into energy to keep them and you firing. Some cells, like nerve cells only have a few mitochondria, others like muscles have thousands and require a lot of energy.

Munching The Calories

Muscle is what is known as active tissue so it really munches its way through the calories. Fat cells, on the other hand are generally more than a little happy to store energy on your hips and bum until they are called into action. So if you want to wake up those fat cells, you have to maintain, or even better gain muscle mass. Starvation studies indicate that parallel losses of lean muscle mass and fatty tissue leave subjects with the same percentage of body fat after weeks of starvation. The metabolic rate diminishes as the percentage of lean muscle mass reduces because the body requires far more energy to move lean muscle than to move fat. Fatty tissue is an energy source and does not require energy to move but if you have a larger percentage of muscle mass not only is movement easier, but you require more energy to do it. This is why exercise is so important in achieving and maintaining a healthy, lean body.

The body requires far more energy to move lean muscle than to move fat.

Many women are afraid of building muscle as they fear it will make them look big, muscular and manly. The reality is that women are just not equipped to build big muscles like men. Levels of the hormone, *testosterone* play a significant role in muscle growth and women only have about a tenth of the amount men do. Hence the reason men can bulk up much more quickly and why they tend to carry less fat than women. All the extra energy-munching their muscles do allows them to consume more calories before the excess is dumped in their fat stores. Many, but certainly not all female bodybuilders use a variety of hormone therapies to achieve the bulked-up muscles they need for competition which generally lead to health problems in the long term for some.

It is a great deal easier to lose muscle than it is to gain it. If you have ever been hospitalised for a spell or injured and unable to move around much you will know that only too well. Muscle wastage occurs very quickly and regaining muscle strength after such an episode can be a long, slow process. So, even if you embark on an exercise programme and for one reason or another you begin to gain more muscle than you are want, alterations to your exercise programme will ensure you lose the bulk you don't like fairly quickly and you can continue to work on the body perfect.

As we age, we naturally begin to lose muscle mass and often gain weight but a comprehensive exercise programme can keep our muscles active and when they are active their mitochondria work flat out. They keep munching on the calories and keep burning up the fat. And it's not just the muscles you see when you look at your body in the mirror that are important (skeletal muscle tissue) but also the ones you can't see (cardiac muscle tissue that forms the bulk of the wall of your heart and smooth muscle tissue that is located in the walls of hollow internal structures such as blood vessels, the stomach, your intestines and bladder). Muscle is a serious player when it comes to physical health and whilst the expression 'use it or lose it' is generally linked to keeping your brain sharp, it applies equally to muscles.

Muscle Drives your Metabolism

Healthy and strong muscles raise our metabolic rate allowing us to burn more calories even when we are not actively working them. We can learn a lot from sport science. Historically, bodybuilders used all sorts of drugs, stimulants and combinations of both to build muscle and lose fat to achieve the *shredded* look required for competition. Similarly, professional athletes embarked on extreme and often drastic regimes to give them the competitive edge. Fortunately, the last twenty years have seen huge changes, important regulation of performance-enhancing aids and an altogether healthier approach to winning gold. Major research into how the human body achieves the physical and nutritional strength, the mental determination and the focus to shave a millisecond off a hundred metre sprint or a day or two off an assault on Everest have revealed a plethora of fascinating studies. The results of these studies have a major impact on how we all perform from day to day whether we intend to push ourselves and take part in a physically challenging charitable event or we just want to get fitter, healthier and minimise fat.

This is predominantly a book about getting the nutritional edge and understanding how, when and why the foods we consume can either add to our waistlines or reduce them, but it would in no way be complete if the deserved respect was not shown to those who work tirelessly to augment our understanding of the most up to date methods of busting fat, with the aid of regular exercise. They know we don't want to spend hours in the gym doing

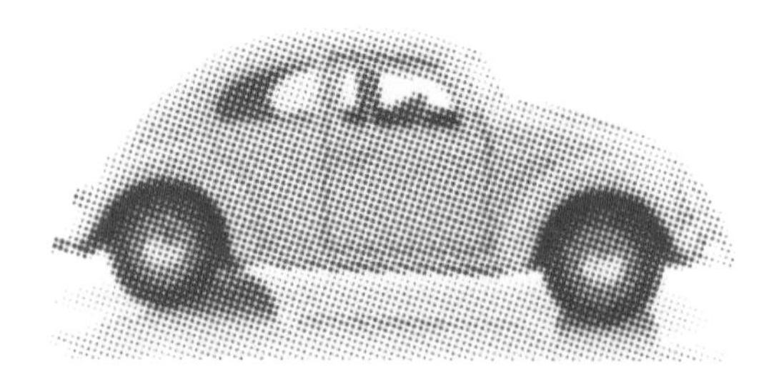

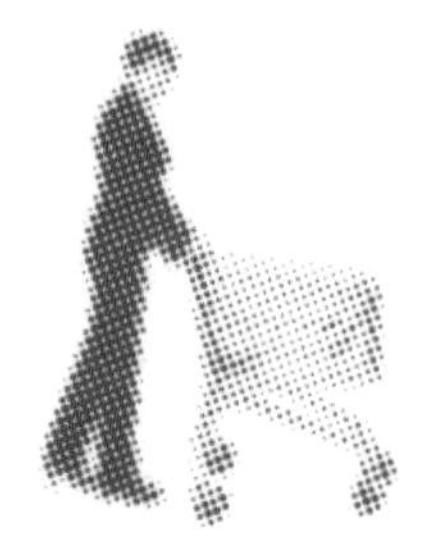

the same old routine, they also appreciate that we are probably short of time and total dedication is tough. As with nutrition, confusion reigns, but there are a few themes emerging which you may wish to consider if you are seriously committed to building muscle to bust fat.

If you want to see great and long-lasting results from the following well-researched exercise/nutrition combination to find the fit, lean and toned body you know is lurking somewhere under those excess pounds of flesh, you may wish to delve more deeply into the science. If so, read some of the many studies available, buy a book that covers this type of programme in detail or enlist the services of a personal trainer who practices these principles.

Here are the bones of how it works:-

Resistance Training. To increase muscle while shedding body fat in the most time-efficient way, quality over quantity is the key. You train hard but for a shorter time and fat burning is accelerated because there is an increased secretion of both *growth hormone* and *noradrenalin*, the hormones that help to mobilise fat stores and use fat for fuel. More calories are expended both during the intense workout and because your BMR (basal metabolic rate) is increased for many hours after you have finished training - that's when the fat burning kicks in.

By using dumbbells, exercise machines, your own body weight, bottles of water, elastic tubing, ankle and wrist weights or exercise bricks, muscles are strengthened by pitting each group against a force (resistance). To develop a muscle you must work all the fibres within it which means pushing them to their limit for short periods of time, resting them briefly then repeating the process. You work with a weight that is heavy enough so that the last few repetitions become difficult to perform. This is not the kind of exercise where you chat to a friend while you workout. It requires concentration and determination. When a muscle is overloaded, lactic acid is produced causing the *burn* in the muscle that ultimately leads to muscular fatigue – you have to push past that sensation and ensure your mind doesn't give up before your body. The rest between repetitions enables the lactic acid to be flushed from the bloodstream, allowing the muscles to be refreshed before working them again.

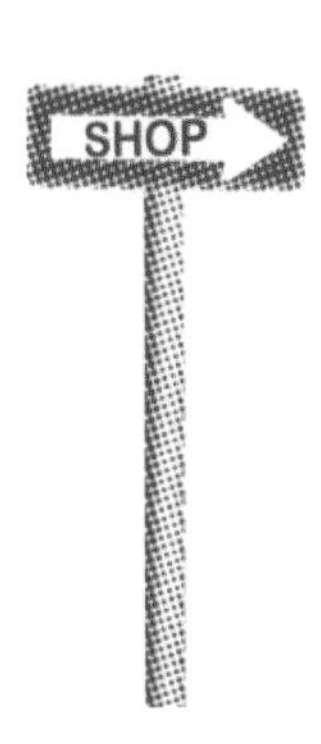

Recommendations vary but generally 30-40 minutes, three times a week is a good goal. To allow the muscles to repair and regenerate 48hrs should be allowed between sessions. This enables protein synthesis to take place (the process by which the body repairs muscle tissue) preventing injury.

And it's never too late to start.

In one study of elderly men and women (average age 87) who lifted weights three times a week for ten weeks, muscle strength increased by a staggering 113% on average. This improvement in strength enabled them to walk 12% faster than before, climb 28% more stairs and lose excess body fat.

Interval Training. Whilst resistance training is the most effective for fat burning for many hours after a workout, it should be coupled with aerobic exercise for a number of reasons. The cardiovascular system becomes more efficient at delivering oxygen to working muscle, delaying the lactic acid build-up which allows you to train at a higher level of intensity. Aerobic exercise also expands the network of blood vessels that allow nutrients to be absorbed into body tissues and the more capillaries we have the better the body becomes at utilising the nutrients for muscular repair. This expanded network of blood vessels also helps to clear waste products, particularly carbon dioxide from the food burning process. Efficient exchange of oxygen and nutrients in and carbon dioxide and waste out is paramount for fit and healthy body tissue.

In addition, the mitochondria (the energy factories) expand in size and number and require more energy. Once they have used up the glycogen (the stored glucose within the muscle cells and the liver), they call on the fat cells to release energy. Interval training provides significant benefits over steady state exercise and is more effective at burning fat because as with resistance training, the fat burning is prolonged after activity. This type of training involves intense effort for one minute followed by less intense effort for between one and four minutes. During the intense phase the lactic acid builds up quickly and during the less intense phase it is cleared from the blood and oxygen stores are replenished. This is repeated multiple times.

Here's an example

If you are a jogger, run as fast and as hard as you can for one minute then reduce your speed to a steady jog for between one and four minutes. Keep repeating until your 30 minutes is up. The same applies to rowing, cycling, swimming, skipping, using a mini trampoline or whatever gets your heart pumping. If you are on the treadmill in the gym, turn the knob to as fast as you can cope with for one minute then turn the speed down to a manageable jog for four minutes. A mere five repetitions and your 30 minutes of cardio are done. As you get fitter you can reduce the number of minutes between the intense phases to two minutes during the middle section of your workout.

Resistance training for 30 minutes on Monday, Wednesday and Friday (or Tuesday, Thursday and Saturday) and Interval Training for 30 minutes on the other three days with one day of rest suits many peoples' timetables, but you may prefer to do both in a one hour workout only three times a week (with one rest day between each). So which should you do first? Resistance followed by Interval appears to have the edge.

Since the body's preferred energy source is glucose that's what we should target first. Resistance Training does that. The body uses the glucose from recently consumed carbohydrates in the bloodstream followed by the stored glucose in the muscles and liver when we perform any type of anaerobic exercise. **Resistance Training is anaerobic** – it uses minimal oxygen and as fat can only be burned in the presence of oxygen the fat cells won't be mobilised into releasing their energy stores until after we stop. By the time we embark on the Interval Training, glycogen stores are pretty well used up and because Interval Training is aerobic (uses lots of oxygen) the body will have to call on the fat stores for energy. And, because of the intensity of both sessions the body will continue to burn calories for hours afterwards, requiring fat stores to continue providing some or much of that energy.

For fat loss, a combination of the following principles appears to reap the greatest rewards:-

- Resistance training (30 minutes every 2 days).
- Interval training (30 minutes every 2 days).
- Rest days (1 day a week if you do the above on separate days or 4 days a week if you combine the two).
- Eating below your recommended calorie base 3-4 days a week.
- Re-feeding to avoid metabolic slowdown every 4 days.

Eating below your recommended calorie base. This does NOT mean cutting calories drastically or endless counting. A very simple method is to take your body weight and multiply by 16. It's not 100% accurate but if you are carting a load of fat around that you want to get rid of, it's a good place to start. So if you are ten stone (140 lbs x 16) your current calorie recommendation is around 2240kcals per day. Start by reducing your intake by between 300 and 500 kcals per day. Remember you are trying to keep the fat burning furnace firing and if you cut too many calories too quickly your body will go into *preservation mode* and turn down the flame resulting in you burning less calories and hitting a plateau. Additionally, those muscles you are trying to develop and strengthen with your resistance training are a ready source of fuel when your body is short of energy and will happily give up their stores resulting in weakening your muscles rather than preserving or building them. **You have to feed muscles not starve them.** Only when they are strong and active will they continue to call on fat cells to release energy and shrink in the process.

The pros and cons of calorie counting have already been discussed and the importance of what, when and how you eat should be crystal clear by now. When you devise your own *Fat Loss Plan* you will be reducing your intake of the calories that make no sense biochemically and you will be feeding your metabolism and your hormones to ensure they don't slow you down. This means you can embrace the Resistance/Interval training programme with confidence. However, if you decide to go for the *2 Weeks in the Fast Lane* route outlined in the next chapter *Shrink the Fat Cells not the Brain Cells* which involves a greater daily reduction in calories and embark on a Resistance/Interval Training programme simultaneously you will have to make a couple of alterations to your eating and re-feed every few days.

Re-feeding. What re-feeding basically means is increasing the number of calories you consume every few days so that the body doesn't think there's a *famine* looming and slow down metabolism to compensate. If you are demanding the level of energy required for an exercise programme such as that outlined above, your body will begin to realise that there simply isn't enough food to cope. But it takes a few days for this situation to occur, so by re-feeding every few days the body keeps burning fat for fuel and helping you shed pounds. Scientific evidence of how this works is scant but as mentioned previously, we are likely to hear a lot more about *calorie shifting* over the next few years. Some fitness professionals use this method, often with great success, so why wait for the green light from all sides - do it now and look forward to a result.

If you are adopting the six days a week workout programme, alternating your Resistance and Interval training with one day off, you should re-feed every fourth day. It doesn't matter which day but if you are going for the three days a week combination of the two with four days off, still re-feed every fourth day but try to ensure that it is a day when you are working out - a day here of there is not vital.

Stick with the eating plan recommended in the *2 Weeks in the Fast Lane* but add one of the recommended re-feed extras every fourth day.

Unfit or Unused to Exercise? Don't worry, the principles of Resistance and Interval training apply no matter where you start. Resistance Training is all about introducing some weights into your life and if you want to start with a couple of cans of baked beans you will still be creating the force and within a couple of weeks you can raise your game and seek out the litre bottles of water. From there it's all uphill. Similarly, Interval Training is all about moving as fast as you can manage for one minute followed by four minutes of slowing the pace. Walking is a great way to start – brisk for one minute, less intense for four. As you get fitter, your body will get acclimatised and you can push the intensity. Remember small changes make the difference.

Other Forms of Exercise. Yoga, Pilates, Swiss Ball, T'ai Chi, Kick-boxing etc. There are so many choices and many if not all of them are good for our health, our heart, our posture, our energy levels and our mood. However, when it comes to prompting the body to use fat stores for energy, a combination of aerobic and anaerobic exercise coupled with an energy-rich diet has definitely prompted the most research. Whatever you choose to do, make sure you build muscle whilst minimising fat gain - work those muscles and push yourself.

Additional Tactics

- When you go to the supermarket, park in the corner of the car park furthest away from the door so you have further to walk both ways (the heavier the shopping bags the more muscle you build!)
- When parking in a multi-storey car park, go straight up to the top level and take the stairs both ways.
- If you are a smoker and you go out of the office for a cigarette break, don't just stand outside and chat to other smokers – walk round the block.
- When you take the kids to the park, don't just stand and watch them, go on the swings with them or run around like they do.
- When you have the dog on the lead, try and walk at the dog's pace rather than training it to walk at yours.
- Don't take the lift unless you have loads to carry.
- Even if you live or work on the top floor, take the stairs for at least two or three floors then the lift for the remainder (and NEVER take the lift down unless you are in a frantic rush).
- Don't buy biscuits, crisps, pastries etc. at the supermarket and keep them in the house. If you really need a treat, walk to the local shops to get it and at least that way you are getting some extra exercise.
- Have more sex! Not only is it a great de-stressor but it burns up the calories (the more energetic, the more calories!)

Part 3. Chapter Sixteen

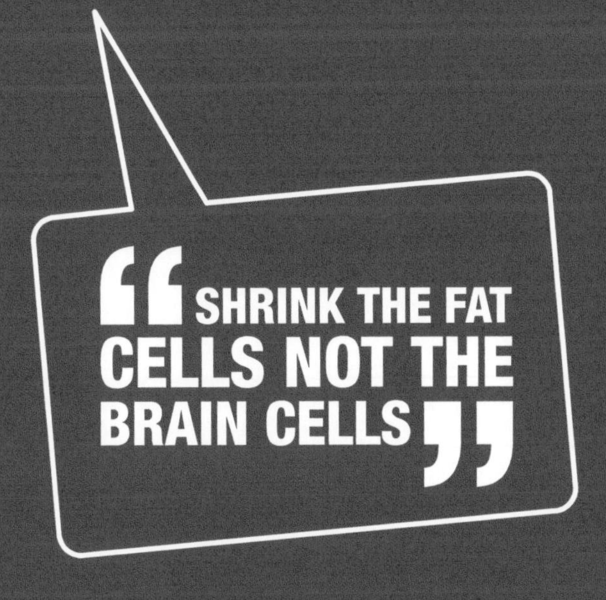

When you gain fat you are not gaining new fat cells, you are just expanding the ones you already have – think of a balloon gradually filling with water!

So should you accept that the only way to shed fat for good is to change your eating habits for good and accept that it's going to be a slow, but ultimately healthier and more successful process? No. You can change your eating habits in a few weeks if you really want to and see some great results that can spur you on to changing a few more. But it's almost impossible if you are constantly tired and hungry, so you have to feed your brain to zap the fat.

The Fat Loss Plan works because you tailor it to your tastes, lifestyle and preferences. There are no hard and fast rules to break because as you create your own diet you address your own needs and prioritise. You don't burden yourself with a host of restrictions.

If however, time is short and there's a red carpet event looming and a speedier result is required, you can get on the right road for a couple of weeks by following the *2 Weeks in the Fast Lane Plan* in this chapter. It's not a detox or a crash diet, it doesn't restrict calories or leave you short of goodness and it's not depressing, distressing, demotivating, demoralising or destructive.

But unlike *The Fat Loss Plan*, there are a few rules

- You have to make it a priority.
- You have to eat something every 2-3 hours.
- You have to start it on any day of the week other than a Monday.
- You have to bin the *white stuff* and only include energy-dense starchy carbohydrates before 6pm.
- You have to get half an hour's physical activity into your day.
- You have to drink water every 2-3 hours.
- You have to keep it simple.

If you want to lose the fat you see in the mirror that has forced you into buying a bigger size or two, you have to convince those fat cells to give up their stores. Women have around 34 billion fat cells and men have around 25 billion and after puberty the number doesn't change much. When you gain fat you are not gaining new fat cells, you are just expanding the ones you already have – think of a balloon gradually filling with water. They can become 5 to 6 times their size so to lose fat you have to get them to shrink and stay shrunk.

Why should you make it a priority? Convincing your body to use fat stores for energy in super-quick time requires careful manipulation of the types of foods you eat so you have to treat it as a project and focus.

Why should you eat something every 2-3 hours? To keep the fat burning furnace firing all day, every day and to ensure you body swerve the energy dips and the cravings. When you are tired and hungry resolve takes a dive.

Why should you start on any day other than Monday? Failed dieters often start a diet on a Monday and see the weekend as an opportunity to pig out before the deprivation starts – hardly a recipe for success. Also, you may have noticed that Monday is the only day of the week that seems to attract negative adjectives like blue, gloomy and depressing. Why risk it? Do your planning and shopping at the beginning of the week, get organised and start midweek instead.

Why should you bin the white foods? They are an instant but short-lived energy source, provide few nutrients and don't fill you up for long. They raise the level of glucose in the bloodstream too quickly and in an effort to regain the necessary balance the sugars are shipped off for immediate use or stored in the liver, muscles and fat cells until required. If you want the fat cells to shrink you can't afford to give them the opportunity to expand their storage facilities. They have to be badgered into releasing their stores to provide energy. Keeping the sugar level balanced by eating colourful nutrient-rich foods can help to achieve this; white foods make it a whole lot harder.

Why should you avoid energy-dense starchy carbohydrates after 6pm? Because they provide energy during the day when you are active but can leave you feeling bloated and uncomfortable at bedtime. They may also promote fat storage through the night (the jury is still out on this one at time of publication but why risk it?)

Why should you get half an hour's physical activity into your day? Because working muscles need lots of energy (20-50 times more than they do at rest) so the fat stores are forced into action yet again. And if you get physical first thing

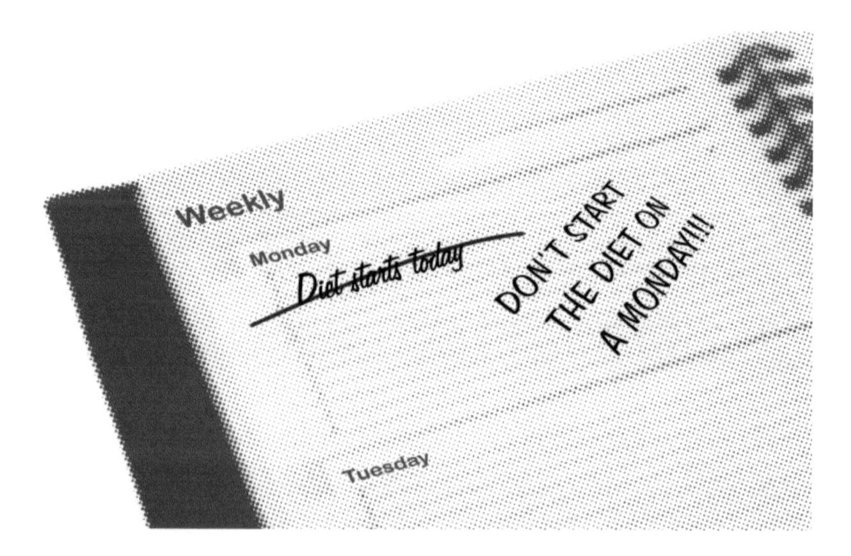

in the morning you fat burn more efficiently for as much as 8 hours afterwards (some suggest it may be as much as 24hrs).

Why should you drink water every 2-3 hours? Because every chemical reaction that takes place in the body 24/7 from extracting nutrients from food to encouraging fat burning needs water to get a result.

Why should you keep it simple? Contrary to the spin surrounding some diets, losing fat is not easy, effortless or care-free. You have to commit. Whilst the debate rages on, many successful dieters agree that too much choice can be a major stumbling block in the early stages. This plan combines maximum nourishment with minimum choice to ensure compliance and success rather than confusion and frustration. Studies show that while extensive choices are initially appealing, subsequent satisfaction and motivation are more often achieved when choice is reduced but variety predominates.

So what do you have to do?

- Get up half an hour earlier and get physical for 30 minutes.
- Skin brush before your shower and eat fruit and drink only juiced fruit/smoothies and still or sparkling water until late morning.
- If you need a hot drink have fresh black coffee, black, green, red bush or herb (but not fruit) tea before or after your late morning snack without milk or sugar.
- Have a late morning snack.
- Have soup and salad around lunchtime.
- If you need another hot drink follow the recommendations above.
- Have a mid afternoon snack.
- Have a light meal around dinner time with no energy-dense starchy carbohydrates.
- Have a small bedtime snack at least 30mins before you go to bed (only if you are really hungry or you find you are waking up in the wee small hours and can't get back to sleep).

1. Get Physical

Re-read the last chapter on exercise, *Your Body is Made of Moving Parts, so*

Move Them to get the latest fat burning exercise combination into your life. Half an hour a day, six days a week – can't be that hard! **Important**: If you adopt the exercise strategy, add some re-feed extras (see end of chapter) into your diet every fourth day to ensure your body is less likely to see your reduced daily calorie intake as a prompt to move into metabolic slowdown and limit fat burning.

2. Skin Brush

Lightly brushing the skin with a dry brush or loofah stimulates the circulation, removes dead skin cells and promotes elimination. Start brushing at your feet and brush towards the heart, then brush from the fingertips up to the shoulders and toward the heart (don't forget the soles of your feet and the palms of your hands). Use small strokes and a gentle pressure - you're not brushing the dog. Avoid the face and neck area and any damaged or bruised skin. Jump into the shower and have a good rinse to get rid of the dead skin cells before soaping. If you are brave enough you can turn the shower to cold (but not freezing) for a few minutes before you dry off to encourage your body to launch into a bit more fat burning to keep warm. If you have an ongoing health condition or are on medication, check with your doctor before considering this rude awakening!

3. Get Fruity

There are a host of reasons why permanent weight loss is such a struggle but a sluggish or inefficient digestive system is one of the most common obstacles. Fruits provide a quick energy source and are bursting with nourishment but when consumed with other foods they can cause havoc for some. By being trapped in the stomach for too long they undergo fermentation which can not only upset the digestive process of other foods but also reduce the nutritional value of the fruit. When you eat them on their own and on an empty stomach they take a mere 30 minutes to pass through the stomach and while reaping all their cleansing and nourishing benefits you avoid possible bloating, flatulence or intestinal irritation that you may be all too familiar with.

Before and after your 30 minutes of exercise and every hour thereafter through to late morning (11.30/noon) have fresh fruit, juiced fruits and fresh fruit smoothies. Select from any of the following, make sure you don't add any proteins or fats (watch out for yoghurt in shop-bought smoothies), go for plenty of variety and wait until late morning before you have your regular cup of tea/coffee.

Fresh fruits straight from the tree/bush

Keep the peel on where possible and give them a good scrub before eating whole or chopping, slicing or dicing. Aim for as much colour as possible throughout the morning and be generous with your portions.

Fresh Fruit Juices

Citrus fruits are born to be juiced. Half a few oranges and get as much as you can out of them (an electric or battery operated citrus press is a cheap and highly effective bonus here). Add lemon, lime, mandarin, tangerine, Clementine and grapefruit to the mix to ring the changes.

Smoothies

All you need is a blender and you're good to go. Sling a few ice cubes and a teacup of water into the blender then add fruits of choice. Berries, cherries (if you can be bothered to stone them), melon, peaches and nectarines, kiwi, tropical fruits like mango, papaya, pineapple, passion fruit and pawpaw, bananas, apples, pears, apricots, plums, grapes, figs, tomatoes (yes, they are a fruit) and of course citrus fruits all blend well – experiment and find your favourite combinations. Bags of frozen fruits are great for smoothies if you don't have time to chop, peel and slice. Strain the juice through a sieve before drinking if you don't like the seedy/gritty bits and add more water if it's too thick and gloopy. Don't down them in one go, sip them slowly and savour the flavours.

Juices

If you already own a juicer, get it out of the cupboard and go for it. You lose a whole lot less of the goodness of the fruits (vitamins, minerals and fibre) when you juice them. Sip them slowly while you are cleaning the machine or pop the juice in a thermos and sip throughout the morning. If you don't have a juicer, see if you can find a juice bar near your work or home and test a few of their fruit combinations but remember; only fruits, no added extras.

Bottled Juices + Smoothies

These provide the least amount of goodness as they have been processed to allow them a few days shelf life, but there are plenty out there that have been sympathetically produced to provide you with as fresh a juice as possible. Generally speaking, price is a good guide - the more expensive they are, the more goodness has been retained and because they are less processed they don't have a long shelf life. You will often find them discounted because their 'use by' date is perilously close – grab them.

4. Have a hot drink if you need it

If you usually have coffee or tea in the morning, you may be struggling by late morning. Now is the time to have your cuppa. Choose good quality black coffee from ground beans, black, green, red bush or herb (not fruit) tea before or after your late morning snack and don't add milk or sugar.

5. Have a late morning snack

Choose one of the following:-

- Small pack of unsalted nuts (no dried fruit).
- Cold, cooked chicken leg or breast (skin removed), a couple of tomatoes and a small handful of fresh nuts.
- Couple of oatcakes spread with tinned, mashed salmon topped with cucumber slices.
- A tray or pack of raw baby vegetables with a small pot of hummus.
- A tray or pack of raw baby vegetables with a small pot of guacamole.
- Bowl of mixed olives with feta cheese cubes or olives stuffed with anchovies or almonds.
- 3 bean salad from the 'deli' section of most supermarkets (or make your own).

6. Get Soupy (+ have a small salad)

It's filling, it's fast, it's nutritious and it's widely available. Have a bowl or mug of soup around lunchtime every day. You can also have soup as your late morning or mid afternoon snack or in the evening if time is the enemy or you are going out. If you do opt for soup for your evening meal occasionally or

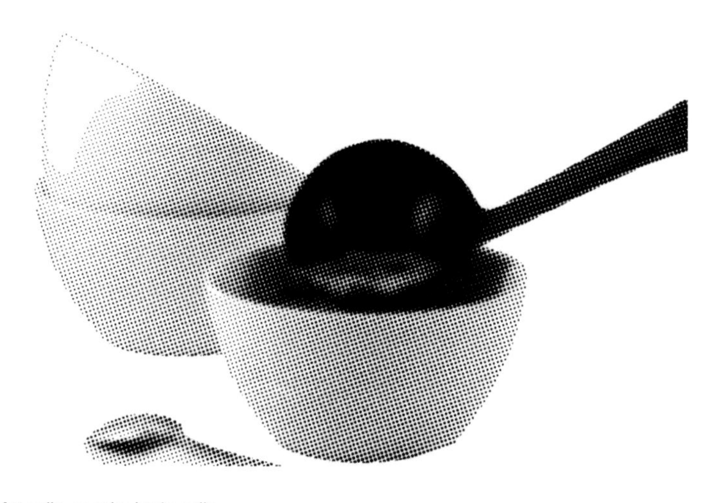

within 4 hours of going to bed, ensure that it is a vegetable, meat, poultry or fish combination with no starchy carbohydrates included (rice, barley, beans, lentils, noodles etc.) Also, experiment with chilled soups if we are having a rare, but welcome heat wave.

Home Made Soups

If you can find the time, these are the healthiest option as you know exactly what's going into them and you can put as few or as many ingredients in as you wish. Experiment with the recipes in chapter 19, *A Few Random Recipes* (and remember to leave out the starchy carbohydrates if you are having a bowl after 6pm).

Ready Made Soups

There are so many varieties available that you could have three different soups a day, seven days a week for at least a month and never have the same one twice. However, there are a great many that are high in fat, salt or sugar (or all three), so label reading is vital. Head for the vegetabley, meaty, fishy, beany ones and body swerve the creamy ones. Be particularly vigilant about packet and tinned soups and remember the important numbers.

Look at the *per 100g* column rather than the *per serving* column and follow the guidelines:-

Spot the sugar – where it says *Carbohydrates: of which sugars*, 10g is high, 2g is low. Aim for a maximum of 4g.

Spot the saturated fat – where is says *Fats: of which saturates*, 5g is high, 1g is low. Aim for a maximum of 2g.

Spot the salt – where it says *Salt or Salt equivalent*, 1.5g is high, 0.3g is low. Aim for a maximum of 0.6g.

Spot the sodium – where it says *Sodium*, 0.5g is high, 0.1g is low. Aim for a maximum of 0.2g

Super Quick Soup

A spoonful of miso paste or a sachet of miso soup dissolved in boiling water is not only warming and tasty but very nutritious and can keep hunger pangs at bay. Same goes for a mug of *Marigold Swiss Vegetable Bouillon*. Keep a tub handy and opt for the low salt version. You can also combine the two. There are scores of quick soups and cuppa soups on the supermarket shelves but many of them are scarily salt-ridden. Again, check the label. However, if you are following the recommended eating plan and adding herbs and spices to your food for added flavour instead of salt, your salt intake should reduce drastically so your soup choice needn't be the enemy. Just keep an eye on it and follow the salt and sodium guidelines above.

Have a Small Salad

You will find a plethora of suggestions for cold and hot salads in chapter 14, *Lots of 'Eats'*. If you opt for a bought/ready made salad, bin the little pack of salad dressing and replace with a mix of olive, nut or seed oil and a squirt of lemon/lime juice

7. Have a hot drink if you need it

Follow the recommendations above before or after your mid afternoon snack and ring the changes.

8. Have a mid afternoon snack

Choose one of the following:-

- Small pack of mixed, unsalted nuts and seeds (no dried fruit).
- Couple of brown Ryvita with chopped boiled egg mixed with natural live yoghurt and chopped herbs.
- A tray or pack of raw baby vegetables with a small pot of natural cottage cheese.
- A tray or pack or raw baby vegetables with a small pot of salsa.
- A cold boiled egg and a couple of slices of cooked ham.
- A couple of sticks of celery filled with nut butter (almond, cashew, hazelnut, macadamia – not peanut).
- A grain bar – the *Food Doctor* and *Gillian McKeith's* are *good choices* (go for the ones without dried fruit).

NB – buy omega 3-rich eggs whenever possible. The hens that lay these eggs are fed on a diet rich in seeds that provide the essential omega 3 fats that help to promote fat burning - and they taste great.

9. Have a light meal around dinner time

This is the time of the day to say no to energy-dense starchy carbohydrates. The combination of a decent portion of good quality protein, some essential fats and plenty of vegetables provide a filling meal that gives your body everything it needs to rest, repair and fat burn all night.

If you are only able to fit your half hour of exercise into the early evening and usually have your meal afterwards, you can add a cupful of brown rice, barley, couscous, beans or lentils, a baked sweet potato or sweet potato chips (scrub, don't peel and cut into generous chips, paint with olive oil and bake in a moderate oven until crispy round the edges and succulent within).

Choose one of the following:-

- A steamed skinless turkey or chicken breast topped with pesto or olive paste.
- A poached salmon fillet or salmon steak painted with *Worcestershire Sauce.*
- Grilled white fish fillets topped with lemon juice and a spoonful of warmed tomato salsa.
- A venison fillet or venison steak marinated for at least 10 minutes in olive oil, a couple of splashes of balsamic vinegar and ground black pepper, then grilled.
- A couple of smoked mackerel fillets baked in the oven until hot.
- Half a dozen fresh prawns coated with chilli oil and grilled.
- A 2 egg omelette or frittata with sliced courgettes, mushrooms, peppers, spinach and a few shavings of parmesan cheese.
- Tofu with garlic and ginger – cut firm tofu into cubes and stir fry in a little olive oil mixed with crushed garlic and grated fresh ginger. Add a squeeze of runny honey and top with toasted flaked almonds.
- Beef or soya mince burger – use freshly ground lean beef, minced or soya mince which has been soaked for half an hour as per packet instructions. Add some sea salt crystals, ground black pepper then other spices of choice (cumin, coriander, curry powder, chilli powder etc), plus a few shakes of *Lea & Perrins* or balsamic vinegar. Mould into burger shapes and chill for 20 minutes before grilling. Top with a slice of goats cheese or cheddar towards the end of cooking.

Have at least 3 different steamed, grilled, stir fried or roasted vegetables (not starchy potatoes, root vegetables or corn) and/or a large mixed salad. Top your vegetables or salad with roasted mixed nuts or seeds or mixed bean sprouts and drizzle with nut or seed oil (avocado, sesame, sunflower, pumpkin, walnut, flax, hemp etc.) and a squeeze of lemon/lime juice.

10. Have a bedtime snack

Only if you are really hungry or you find you can't get to sleep or you regularly wake up in the wee small hours and can't get back to sleep. The following food combinations are rich in the amino acid, *tryptophan* which encourages the production of the *sleepy* chemical, *serotonin* plus if your blood sugar is all over the place can help to get the balance right overnight. Have your snack at least 30 minutes before you go to bed. You will probably find after a few days *in the fast lane* you will be sleeping better and it won't be required:-

- A couple of mini oatcakes with nut or seed butter and a couple of slices of cold turkey breast.
- A mug of Green & Black's hot chocolate made with soya milk.
- A small tub of natural cottage cheese with a handful of mixed seeds.
- One egg lightly scrambled on an oatcake.
- A small carton of natural live yoghurt with a swirl of honey.
- 2 or 3 squares of dark chocolate (70% cocoa solids minimum) and a few shavings of parmesan cheese.
- A small plate of porridge made with water and topped with a spoonful of *Manuka* honey.

Re-feed Extras

If you decide to adopt the exercise plan in the last chapter *Your Body is Made of Moving Parts*, add **one** of the following every **fourth** day before 6pm. If your workout can only be fitted in after work you will already be including a portion of energy-dense starchy carbohydrates with your meal as mentioned but feel free to substitute any of the following.

You will find all the recipes at the back of the book:-

- Portion of special brown rice
- Portion of mejadarra
- Portion of dhal
- Portion of special porridge
- Portion of cold oats

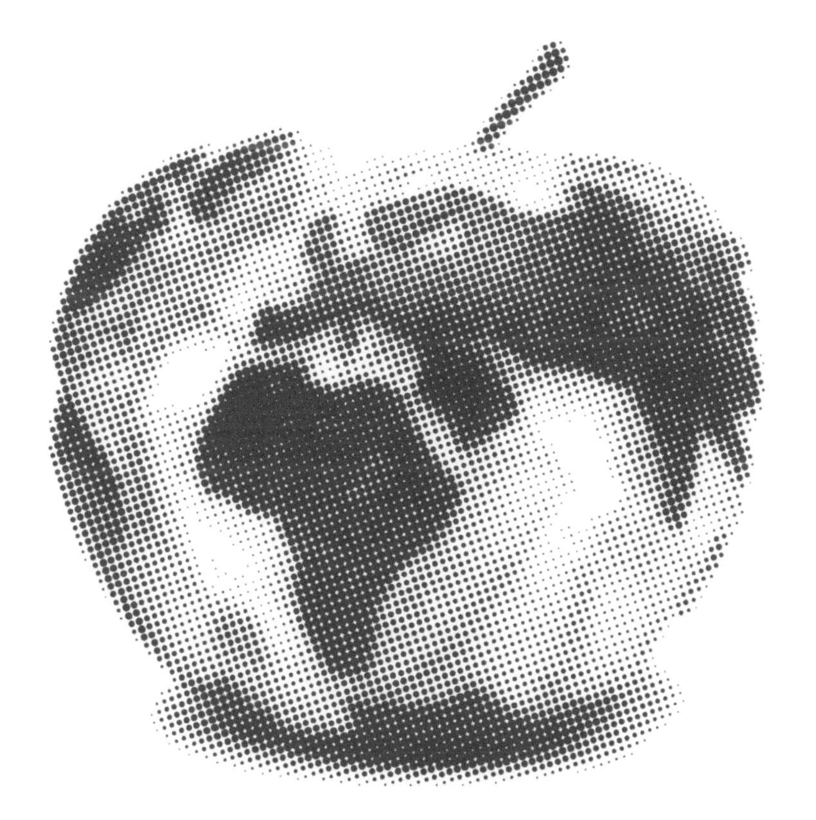

Suggested 7 day plan

IMPORTANT: Whilst soup features daily in this plan, **it is not a liquid diet.** You may wish to substitute soup for your late morning or mid afternoon snack occasionally and even for your evening meal if time is short or you are going out, but don't fall into the trap of **living on fruit juice and soup** day after day for 2 weeks. Variety is the key to successful fat loss.

First thing in the morning

- 30 minutes exercise followed by a large glass of water
- Skin brush and shower

Every hour until late morning (11.30am/noon)

- Fresh Fruits, Juiced Fruits, Fruit Smoothies and Fresh Fruit Juices

Late Morning and Mid Afternoon

- Hot drink

Throughout the day (every couple of hours)

- Still or sparkling water

Day 1

Late Morning	Small pack of unsalted nuts
Lunchtime	Soup and Salad
Mid Afternoon	Ryvita and chopped egg
Evening	Smoked mackerel fillet, vegetables/salad *(and a re-feed extra if you exercise in the evening etc.)*
Bedtime	Oatcakes and turkey slices

Day 2

Late Morning	Oatcakes with tinned salmon and cucumber
Lunchtime	Soup and Salad
Mid Afternoon	Grain Bar
Evening	Chicken or turkey breast, vegetables/salad *(and a re-feed extra if you exercise in the evening etc.)*
Bedtime	Hot chocolate

Day 3

Late Morning	Raw baby vegetables with hummus
Lunchtime	Soup and Salad
Mid Afternoon	Cold boiled egg and ham
Evening	Poached salmon, vegetables/salad *(and a re-feed extra if you exercise in the evening etc.)*
Bedtime	Porridge and honey

Day 4

Late Morning	Cold cooked chicken, tomatoes and fresh nuts
Lunchtime	Soup and Salad
Mid Afternoon	Raw baby vegetables with salsa
Evening	Garlic and ginger tofu, vegetables/salad *(and a re-feed extra if you exercise in the evening etc.)*
Bedtime	Chocolate and Cheese

Day 5

Late Morning	3 Bean Salad
Lunchtime	Soup and Salad
Mid Afternoon	Raw baby vegetables with cottage cheese
Evening	Omelette or frittata, vegetables/salad *(and a re-feed extra if you exercise in the evening etc.)*
Bedtime	Yoghurt and honey

Day 6

Late Morning	Mixed olives with feta cheese or stuffed olives
Lunchtime	Soup and Salad
Mid Afternoon	Small pack of fresh nuts and seeds
Evening	Venison fillet or steak, vegetables/salad *(and a re-feed extra if you exercise in the evening etc.)*
Bedtime	Cottage cheese and seeds

Day 7

Late Morning	Raw baby vegetables with guacamole
Lunchtime	Soup and Salad
Mid Afternoon	Celery sticks with nut butter
Evening	Beef or soya burger, vegetables/salad *(and a re-feed extra if you exercise in the evening etc.)*
Bedtime	Oatcake and scrambled egg

3 Days in the Super-Fast Lane

Are you game for a super-super quick and healthy route to fat loss when time is really short? If you only have a few days and are totally determined, you can live on fresh fruit, nuts and water and you won't go hungry or miss out on essential nutrients. Both fruits and nuts grow on trees and bushes and their roots strike deep into the earth where they take up precious minerals. They also send their limbs high into the space above where, from air and the sun they take in the carbon dioxide that enables them to produce their fabulously nutritious seeds. Between them they supply the body with good levels of the 'Big 6' to keep you nourished daily.

Nuts have had a lot of negative press on the weight management front. Many avoid them, believing them to be fattening – quite the contrary. Nuts are a natural food and rich in many heart-healthy nutrients including monounsaturated and polyunsaturated fats, magnesium, potassium and fibre. In a review of 13 individual studies assessing the effects of nuts on weight, all recorded no increase in weight when nuts were used to replace other foods. Even when nuts were added to an existing diet, all but one study found no tendency toward weight gain. Researchers have suggested that this may be related to the ability of the essential fats in nuts to satisfy the appetite and reduce overall intake of food. There is also evidence as discussed previously, that consuming healthy fats such as those found in nuts, can help the body to burn fat.

This is not for the faint-hearted and under no circumstances should be continued for days on end. The recommendation is three days, but if your schedule is not too manic, you may manage five.

There are, however a few very important points you must address:-

- If you cheat, you won't lose – fruit and nuts are the only foods involved, water is the only drink (still or sparkling).
- Variety is key to gaining the maximum nutrients.
- The better the quality of the produce, the greater the nutritional status so go for the freshest you can find.
- You will undo all your good work and foil your fat burning hopes if you return to your normal eating practices after your *super fast lane experience*, so move immediately onto *The Fat Loss Plan* or the *2 Weeks in The Fast Lane Plan.*
- You may feel a little headachy, lethargic and cold for the first day or perhaps even two if you have been living a life of junk – don't resort to over the counter medication, just drink more water, go to bed earlier (with a hot water bottle and bed socks), luxuriate in a hot bath and add a couple of extra layers of clothing during the day. It will pass and you will start to feel great by day two or three.

Peanuts are not nuts

They are legumes like beans, lentils and peas. They grow in pods on stringy plants on the ground and whilst all legumes are a great source of protein, carbohydrate and fibre, they can be difficult to digest. They play a major role in *The Fat Loss Plan* because of their nutritional prowess but if you are unused to eating them they have to be introduced into your diet slowly and the *3 Days in the Super-Fast Lane Plan* has no room for any foods that take time to get comfortable with.

Instead, get all the other nuts on the planet into your day. Almonds, walnuts, hazelnuts, cashews, pistachios, Brazils, macadamias, pine nuts, chestnuts, pecans – the lot.

Fruit should be eaten on its own on an empty stomach at least one hour before or after the nuts. Water can be drunk at any time of the day, with or without food.

Follow the guidelines in the *Get Fruity* Section of the *2 Weeks in the Fast Lane Plan* and have a combination of fresh fruit, frozen fruit, juiced fruits or smoothies during the day to ensure variety, then choose your nuts wisely to get plenty of protein, essential fats and fibre which will keep you feeling fuller for longer. Salted and roasted nuts are not on the menu here, only fresh nuts in their shells, sold loose or in bags. If they are already shelled, make sure you store them in the fridge to keep them fresh, crunchy and nutrient-rich.

Aim to have fruit or nuts every two hours, but if you start to feel hungry, tired or a bit dazed don't ignore it, just bring your next feed forward. As long as you leave an hour between one snack and the next and sip water throughout the day your body won't see *famine* on the horizon and will efficiently turn your food into energy.

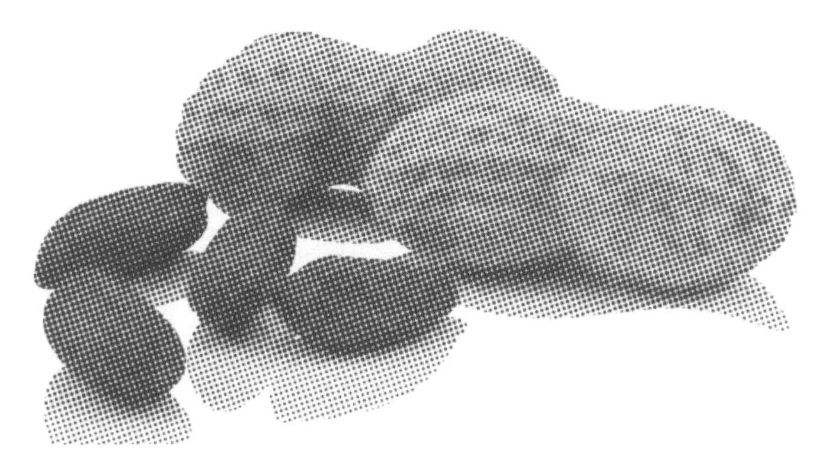

Important. Don't allow more than two hours to go between snacks. If you do, metabolic slowdown may be on the cards.

As far as portions go, it's vital that you enjoy every snack but don't stuff yourself – its only another couple of hours (or less) before you will be eating again so a couple of pieces of fruit, a juice or a smoothie or a couple of handfuls of nuts are all that are required to keep you energised and sharp.

Aim to have your last snack of the day at least 30 minutes before you go to bed and make sure you have water by the bedside to keep you hydrated through the night. You may wish to have a mug of hot water with a couple of slices of fresh lemon first thing in the morning or before bed if you are feeling a bit chilled. Same applies throughout the day.

If you stick this out for 3-5 days and move on to *The Fat Loss Plan* or the *2 Weeks in the Fast Lane Plan* you should not only feel a whole lot more energetic, but you are likely to find that you can get a couple of thumbs between you and the waistband of your favourite skirt or pair of jeans. How much more satisfying is that than merely looking for the needle to take a left turn on the scales? Bin them and press on, you have just made fantastic progress and you are on your way to further fat loss.

And don't forget your half hour of exercise every day – preferably in the morning.

Part 3. Chapter Seventeen

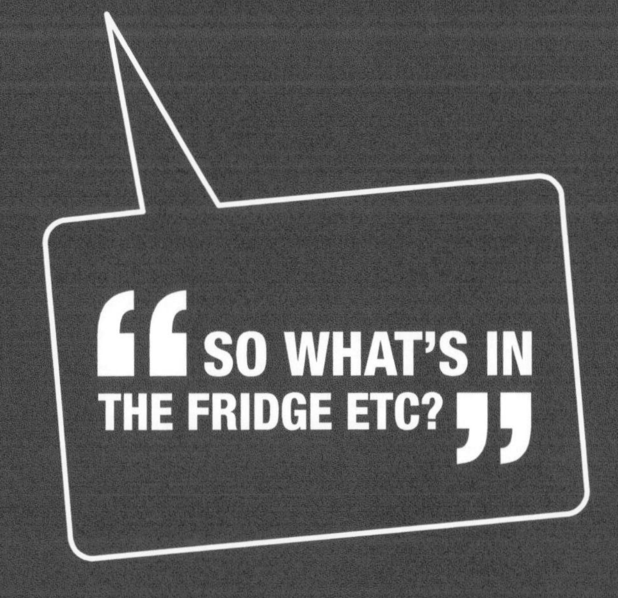

When hunger strikes and you can reach for the biscuit tin – you probably will! But a snack in the handbag is worth its weight in gold.

You Have to be Ahead of the Game!

So how can it go so terribly wrong sometimes? It is really important to have a selection of *good choice* foods and food products within reach at all times.

There is little doubt that when you can reach for the salty snacks or the biscuits – you possibly will!

Mission

Make sure you have lots of *good choice* foods in the following places:-

- IN THE FRIDGE
- IN THE FREEZER
- IN THE CUPBOARD
- IN THE FRUIT BOWL
- IN THE DESK DRAWER
- IN THE GLOVE COMPARTMENT
- IN YOUR HANDBAG/BRIEFCASE

Always

These foods and drinks are all up there at the top of the nutritional class. Try to get as many of them as you can into your daily diet.

Most of the time

All great foods but not a daily requirement.

Occasionally

None of these foods and drinks are off limits but they are definitely *not so good choices* because they are either too rich, too heavy on sugars, salts or fats or just a burden on the body, so give them a wide berth most days and treat them as a 20 option.

174 So what's in the fridge etc.

So what's in the fridge?

Always

- **Eggs** (Columbus, organic or free range) and quails eggs for snacks and speed.
- **Vegetables** (red, green, orange, yellow, purple, white, brown – keep the vegetable drawer full of as much colour as possible. If you are short of preparation time the ready to cook bags, boxes, pouches etc. are still a *good choice).*
- **Salad stuff** – every kind of lettuce, Chinese leaves, chicory, spinach leaves, watercress, rocket, fresh parsley and mixed herbs, fennel, salad onions, mustard cress, baby gem lettuce, celery, chives, cucumber, tomatoes of all shapes and sizes, radishes, sweet peppers.
- **Fresh herbs** – basil, sage, tarragon, dill, oregano, mint or mixed herbs. Add to hot or cold salads, scatter on top of soups, mix into omelettes and frittatas and as a last minute addition to stir fries.
- **Oily Fish** (mackerel, salmon, sardines, anchovies, herring, kippers, trout, fresh tuna, eel, whitebait, swordfish).
- **Other Fish and Shellfish** - go for variety and make friends with your fishmonger if you can't cope with the heads and tails and bones etc (and ask his advice, he's the expert).
- **Nuts** (almonds, Brazils, walnuts, pine nuts, pecans, pistachios, macadamias, hazelnuts, cashews) – keep an eye on the 'sell by' date as they go rancid quite quickly and store in glass jars if you can. Also, if you buy bags of mixed unsalted nuts or nuts and raisins or dried fruits, they will stay fresher and tastier if you keep them in the fridge.
- **Seeds** (flax, linseed, sesame, pumpkin, sunflower, safflower, hemp – also best stored in glass jars).
- **Nut, Seed and Vegetable Oils** (use for cooking, drizzling, spreading, splashing, adding to soups and stews after cooking – DELICIOUS!)
- **Nut and Seed Butters** (use instead of butter) - Pumpkin Seed Butter is particularly scrumptious, even though it looks a bit like green slime!
- **Tofu** (keeps for ages and because it takes up the flavours of the other ingredients is particularly good in stir fries and clear noodley-type soups).
- **Milk and Dairy Products** (go for low fat, skimmed and semi skimmed whenever possible) – milk, best quality butter you can buy/afford, crème fraiche, natural live yoghurt, natural Greek set yoghurt, cottage cheese, quark and fromage frais.
- **Chocolate**-buy the teeny bars of Green & Blacks and when nothing else will do but chocolate, eat one, enjoy it and move on!
- **Dips and Spreads** - hummus, tzatziki, salsa, guacamole, tahini
- **Jars, Bottles and Cartons** – sun dried tomatoes, roasted peppers, artichoke hearts, lemon and lime juice, sugar-free jams and purees,

low sugar peanut butter (crunchy and smooth), horseradish sauce, tomato puree, crushed garlic, pesto, capers, honey, fresh 100% pure fruit and vegetable juices (inc. tomato, carrot and V8)

- **Bean Sprouts**
- **Chilled White Wine**

Most of the Time

- **Chicken and Turkey** – go for free-range, organic birds and cuts wherever possible and ensure you keep an eye on the sell by date. Lean is best, so bin the skin wherever possible
- Rice Milk, Soya Milk, Oat Milk, Nut Milk, Goats Milk
- Game – venison, duck
- Cold cooked meats
- Low Salt/Low Sugar Pasta Sauces
- Bacon Bits and Cubed Pancetta
- Cheese (goats and ewes milk esp.) but also hard cheeses, buffalo mozzarella, ricotta
- Deli Salads – Mixed Beans, Carrot, Couscous, Sun Dried tomatoes etc. (watch out for the amount of sugar in some deli salads)

Occasionally

- Soft and Full Fat Cheeses
- Full Fat Milk and Cream
- Lean Beef and Lamb Cuts
- Good Quality Mayonnaise

So what's in the freezer?

Always

- Frozen Mixed Vegetables
- Frozen Peas/Frozen Spinach
- Frozen Mixed Fruit
- **Frozen Herbs** – coriander, dill, mint, oregano, thyme, tarragon sage etc.
- **Fresh Ginger** – peel, cut into chunks and wrap, then grate from frozen over stir fries, soups and juices before popping back into the freezer
- Sliced Rye and Multigrain Breads
- Tortilla Wraps
- Soups and Stocks
- Frozen Fish and Shellfish

Most of the Time

- **Skinless Chicken, Turkey and Duck Breasts** – go for free-range, organic birds and cuts wherever possible
- Whole Wheat Bagels
- Wholemeal Pizza Bases

Occasionally

- Bacon Bits and Cubed Pancetta
- Lean Minced Lamb and Beef
- Lean Steak
- Lean Lamb Chops
- Bagels, Ciabattas, French breads
- Filo Pastry
- **Muffins, Waffles, Pancakes, Carrot Cake, Banana Cake, Fruit Loaf** (best quality you can afford or homemade)
- **Top Quality Ice Cream and Frozen Yoghurt** (homemade if you have time)

So what's in the cupboard?

Always

- **Grains** – barley, buckwheat, corn, millet, oats, quinoa, rice (brown), couscous
- **Beans** – kidney, haricot, flageolet, pinto, black-eye, lima, chickpeas, soybeans etc. (dried and/or tinned)
- **Lentils** – puy, red, brown, green (dried and/or tinned)
- **Breads** – rye, pumpernickel, wholegrain, Oatcakes, Ryvita, Rye Crackers, Corn Cakes, Rice Cakes, Popcorn (low salt)
- **Olives** – whole green, whole black, stuffed with pimientos, anchovies or almonds
- **Muesli Mix** - low and no sugar
- **Breakfast Cereals** – low and no sugar
- **Teas** – green, herb, fruit and red bush
- **Miso** – granules or paste
- **Tinned Fish** – salmon, crab, tuna, sardines, anchovies, mackerel (best quality for maximum nutrition)
- **Dried Fruits** – prunes, unsulphured apricots, raisins, sultanas, currants, cranberries, apples, mangoes, pears

- Dried Herbs and Spices
- Dried Mushrooms
- Tinned Chopped Tomatoes
- **Salts** – Maldon Flakes, Solo, Lo Salt, Herbamare or crushed dried seaweed
- **Marigold Vegetable Powder** (low salt, for making stocks, sauces and instant soups)

Most of the Time

- Tacos, Nachos, Tortilla Wraps
- Pita Pockets
- **Good Dried Pastas and Noodles** (rice, egg, buckwheat)
- **Black, Green and Red Peppercorns** (for grinding)
- **Red Wine** – particularly Merlot, Cabernet Sauvignon and Chianti
- **Vinegars** - red wine, white wine, cider, raspberry, balsamic
- **Dark and Light Soya Sauce**
- **Mustards** - wholegrain, Dijon and mustard powder
- Tabasco Sauce
- Thai Fish Sauce (nam plah)

Occasionally

- **Heinz Baked Beans** – if you're going to have the sugar-laden variety, they have to be Heinz!
- **Sweet Corn Kernels** – great in salads and soups
- Pretzels
- Blue Corn Tortilla Chips
- Amaretti Biscuits
- Waffle and Pancake Mixes (wholegrain)
- Good Quality Bought Fruit Cake, Carrot Cake, Banana Cake
- Black Tea
- **Good Coffee Beans** (for grinding)
- **Green & Blacks Chocolate Flakes** (for making hot chocolate)
- Tomato Ketchup
- Sweet Chilli Sauce
- Worcestershire Sauce
- Redcurrant Jelly
- Mint Sauce

So what's in the fruit bowl?

Always

- **Fresh Fruits** - variety is the key
- Fresh Tomatoes
- **Squashes** – butternut, acorn, pumpkin
- Sweet Potatoes
- Fresh Dates
- Raw Chestnuts
- Avocados
- Fresh Nuts in their Shells

So what's in the desk drawer?

[If you don't have access to a fridge at work, see if you can lay your hands on an inexpensive wide-necked thermos for the foods that should be kept cool - or just miss them out!]

Always

- An apple with a handful of nuts and seeds
- Raw baby vegetables with hummus, tzatziki, natural yoghurt or salsa
- A few oatcakes, rice cakes, Ryvita or rye crackers
- A banana (to spread on the above)
- Nut or seed butter (to spread on the above)
- *Marigold* vegetable powder and Miso granules or paste for making a quick cup of soup
- Tub of wholegrain cereal (just add low fat milk)
- Fresh nuts and Mixed nuts and raisins
- Nut, Fruit and Seed Bars (no sugar)
- Bowl of mixed berries with shelled pistachios thrown over
- Fruit smoothies (homemade or bought)
- Fruit juice concentrate (just add water)
- Bottle of water
- Low fat natural or set yoghurt with some fresh fruit and a drizzle of honey

Most of the Time

- Cold cooked chicken leg, thigh or breast
- Sliced apple with a handful of mixed nuts and seeds and a chunk of hard cheese
- A cold boiled egg or a few cold boiled quails eggs

- Handful of cherries with slices of goats cheese
- Low salt popcorn, bluecorn tortilla chips, pretzels or organic corn chips
- A few fresh dates stuffed with pistachios

Occasionally

- 3 bean salad from the deli
- Carrot salad from the deli
- Rice salad from the deli
- Slices of fresh melon and parma ham
- Small pack of sushi
- Half an avocado stuffed with fresh prawns or good tinned tuna
- Bowl of mixed olives with feta cheese
- Small bar of Green & Blacks Dark Chocolate

So what's in the glove compartment?

Always

- Fresh Fruit
- Chopped Raw Vegetables
- Fresh Nuts
- Mixed Nuts and Seeds
- Bottle of water
- Mini Oatcakes
- **Banana** - to spread on the mini oatcakes
- **Nut Butter** – to spread on the mini oatcakes
- Fruit Smoothie

Most of the Time

- Dried Fruit
- Mixed Nuts, Seeds and Dried Fruit
- No Sugar or Low Sugar Cereal Bars
- Low Salt Pretzels or corn chips

Occasionally

- **Chocolate** – a small bar of Green & Blacks Dark Chocolate
- Packet of Wine Gums
- Low Salt Vegetable Crisps
- Couple of mini muffins
- Apple and a chunk of hard cheese

So what's in the handbag/briefcase?

Always

- A piece of fruit
- Fresh nuts
- Seed Mix
- Mixed Nuts and Seeds
- Bottle of water

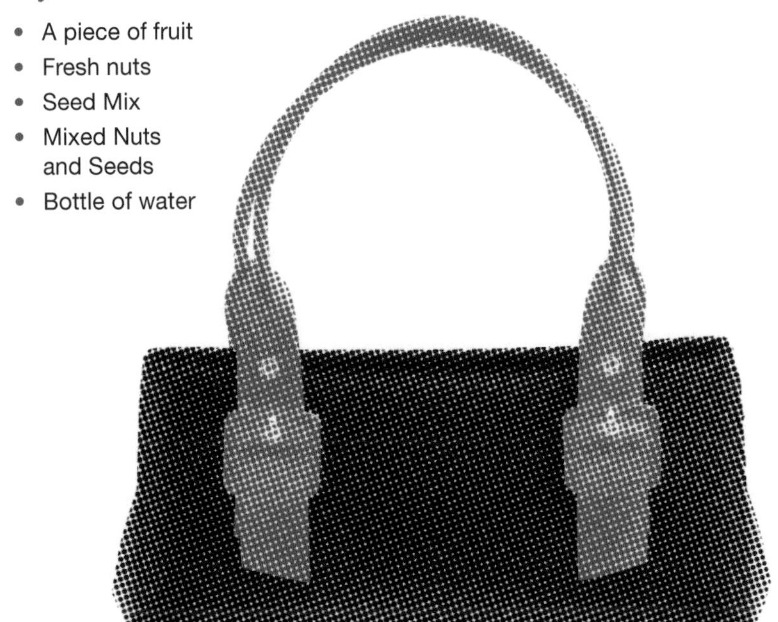

Most of the Time

- **Fruit Slices** – a small pack of freshly sliced pineapple, mango, berries or melon
- Fruit smoothie
- Dried Fruit
- No Sugar or Low Sugar Cereal Bars

Occasionally

- **Chocolate** - small bar of Green & Blacks Dark Chocolate
- Packet of Wine Gums
- Packet of Jelly Babies

Part 3. Chapter Eighteen

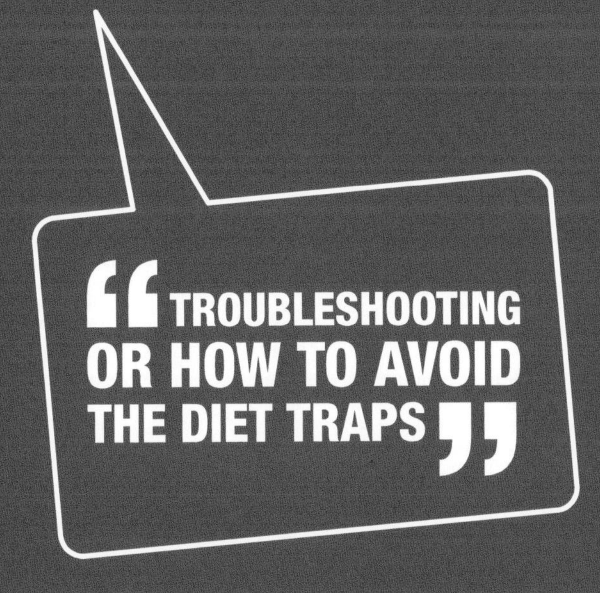

It doesn't have to be about munching on limp salads and sipping water while your mates are gorging on Spaghetti Bolognese and quaffing gallons of Pinot Grigio!

This is without question the biggest stumbling block for anyone trying to lose fat. Foods and drinks that threaten our resolve are around every corner, on every high street, at every café, restaurant, pub, sandwich shop and takeaway. Whilst healthy choices are flagged up on some menus, more often than not they don't tempt the taste buds or fulfil our desire to enjoy the experience of eating and drinking whether we are on our own or with family and friends.

But it doesn't have to be all about cheerless, watery soups and tasteless 'healthy' concoctions. It doesn't have to be about munching on limp salads and sipping water while your mates are gorging on steaming plates of Spaghetti Bolognese and quaffing gallons of Pinot Grigio. *Good choices* don't have to mean dull choices. When you know what to look for, know what to pick from the huge selection on offer and know that some of your favourites don't always have to be on the forbidden list, it can work.

When hunger strikes and you haven't eaten for a number of hours you are at your most vulnerable.

If you are travelling, have a deadline to meet, have to work overtime, haven't had a chance to think about food all day or when domestic or family issues overtake, it's all too easy to forget to eat. Suddenly 4 or 5 hours have elapsed and all that has passed your lips is coffee, tea and a few 'smokes'. This is when good sense goes out the window and comfort food beckons. A bar of chocolate, a packet of crisps, a portion of chips and cheese, a slice of cake – whatever is nearest will do just to get you through the next couple of hours. Worse still, when you get home, meet up with your friends or get to your hotel there is only one thing you want to do - relax with a load of sugary, starchy carbohydrates and possibly a glass or two of your favourite poison. It's reality, it's not unusual and it happens to most of us.

Avoiding The Saboteurs

Troubleshooting on the fat loss front is about being ahead of the game and recognising when and where it can all go wrong. Reminding yourself that *you are eating to lose fat and not starving to gain it* is crucial. Tips on how to avoid the saboteurs and stay on course can be life savers.

Here are the ones to remember

- Stick with the ***small and often plan*** wherever possible. When you are really hungry, are experiencing a blood sugar dip or have allowed too many hours to go by without food you are very likely to devour the nearest snack with scant regard to its nutritional qualities.
- **Plan ahead** whenever possible and ensure you have *good choice* snacks in your handbag/briefcase/glove compartment etc. Just a couple of handfuls of nuts or a chicken leg can quickly tame the hunger monster within.

- Make sure you have a **little protein with every small meal and snack** to slow down the pace at which your food releases its energy-giving nutrients and keep you nourished until your next snack/meal.
- **Include some essential fats** in two or three meals/snacks per day to keep you feeling fuller for longer and keep cravings at bay (nuts, seeds and their oils and butters, oily fish or avocado are tops).
- **Eat energy-dense starchy carbohydrates during the day** but body swerve them after 6pm whenever possible (particularly bread, cereals, potatoes, pasta and rice).
- **Write it down.** This is something people do when money is tight – noting down what we spend on a daily basis for a couple of weeks can be a great tool when we want to cut back on expenditure. The same applies to scribbling down what we eat in a day. If you are honest with yourself and record everything, you quickly see patterns emerging. This allows you not only to take evasive action and avoid the energy dips that lead to poor food choices but also to spot the foods that feature repetitively in your day so you can make a few alterations.
- **Get the portion thing under control.** Use smaller plates, bowls, glasses and mugs, have two starters rather than a starter and main course and order less than you think you can eat when you are out. Have a single sandwich rather than a double in *Pret, Costa, Starbucks* etc., walk past the 2 for 1 offers, avoid 'all you can eat' buffets like the plague and treat the words *mega, super* and *giant* as the enemy. Fat cells have little chance of shrinking if your day is peppered with overly-large portions.
- **Don't keep it a secret.** When you are seriously trying to shed fat it is tempting to keep it to yourself. This is believed to be because we are more than a little nervous about whether we can achieve our goal and admitting defeat sits uncomfortably with most of us. However, it appears that when we have support and encouragement from friends and family the chance of success is much greater. So ignore those that want to sabotage your fat loss goal with comments like "oh, go on, a slice of pizza won't hurt, surely" and spend more time with those who are totally behind you.

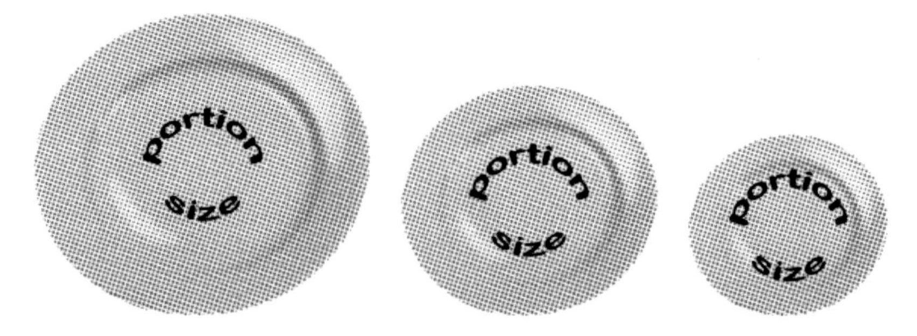

- **Make little changes on a weekly basis.** Clearing the cupboards, fridge and freezer of all the foods you love and regularly buy and heading to the supermarket with a huge list of allowed foods that you may be unfamiliar with and have no idea how to cook only works for the very disciplined or those who are blessed with the time to learn a lot of new tricks. Instead, make one of the above your goal for a week or two then add another.
- **Get physical regularly.** A mere 100 extra calories expended every day can mean up to two stone of weight lost in a year. 20 minutes of brisk walking is one way to achieve this (brisk is roughly 100 steps per minute). Some studies show that just as yo-yo dieting can result in metabolic slowdown and ultimate fat gain so can yo-yo exercising, so do it daily.

Additional Tactics

Most people who lose fat and keep it off have a few tricks up their sleeve – either personal discoveries they have made or habits they have adopted that have helped them to get lean and stay lean. A few have merited some research and analysis, others are just personal coping techniques.

Some could prove to be valuable additions to your quest:-

- When you keep it simple in the early stages you are more likely to stick to your plan.
- Every time you find yourself making excuses, note them down somewhere then work on avoiding those circumstances.
- The hormone that helps to depress appetite appears to be higher in those that get a regular 8 hours sleep. Conversely, the hormone that stimulates appetite can be higher in those that are regularly sleep-deprived so try and get 8 hours a night.
- Going to bed an hour earlier and getting up an hour earlier means you are not tempted to eat late at night and you have time to exercise first thing in the morning.
- Goal setting is one of the greatest success strategies you can employ when it comes to fat loss. Write them down on post-it notes and stick them on the fridge or bathroom mirror, record them on your mobile phone etc. and keep referring back to them.
- Some find that sticking with fruit until late morning makes them feel healthy and focused on their target which results in greater commitment for the rest of the day.
- Eating on the run or in a rush creates stress within the body and turns on the fat storing mechanisms so take your time when you have the time.
- Cutting out or vastly reducing consumption of wheat and/or dairy products can result in significant fat loss and improved digestion for

many. Intolerance to one or the other is on the increase, but cutting them out can be hard, so try one at a time for a couple of weeks, if you can and see how your waistband feels.

- Having a protein shake can quickly satisfy hunger when your day is full on. Don't regard them as meal replacements however and check the label as many of them are loaded with sugar.
- Posting your diet on the internet and sharing your successes and concerns with other bloggers works for some. Others however, end up more confused than when they started!
- Spend time with slim people. Their shopping, cooking and eating habits can reveal a lot about how they stay that way.
- Wearing a pedometer when out walking or jogging has been shown to result in people walking around a mile a day more than those who don't.
- Putting money in a jar/box every time you stick to your daily goal means you can afford to give yourself a reward from time to time – preferably not food!

Other slightly more unusual ploys include brushing your teeth or sucking an ice cube before you eat so you eat less, wearing blue tinted glasses as blue food is not as enticing as other colours and some successful dieters even throw out all their 'fat' clothes, but that may prove pricey!

Taking pictures on your mobile phone of all the food and drink you consume in a day and transferring them to the computer to build a 'visual food diary' can be VERY revealing! A number of studies where people were filmed over a 24/48 hour period then asked to report on exactly what they ate and drank indicate that we typically under-report our consumption by 300-400kcals - even when we know we are being watched! A visual reference may be an excellent route to overcoming this type of 'food amnesia'. Worth a try.

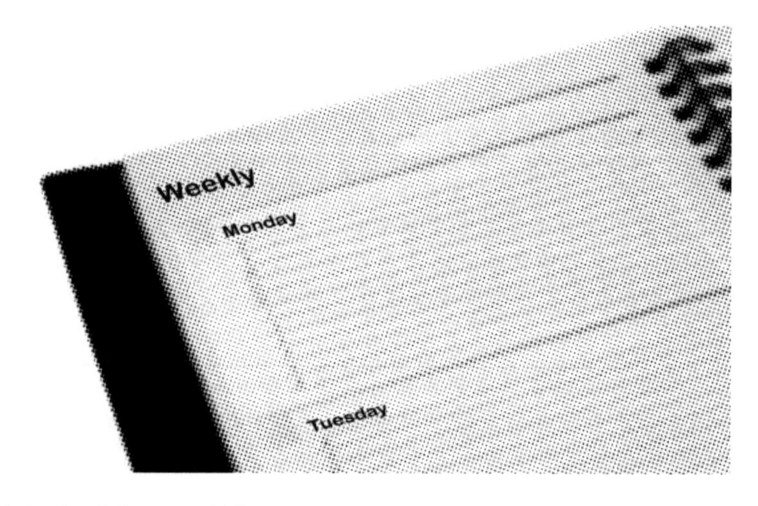

Part 3. Chapter Nineteen

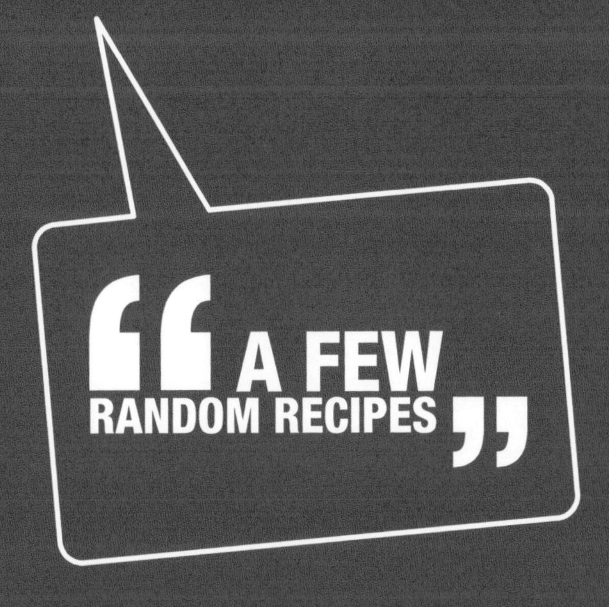

Become a Delia, Jamie or Gordon in no time!

Great Soup Every Time

Once you have made a tasty soup base you can use it to create your own *soup of the day* every day – just remember to add fresh vegetables, some good quality protein, starchy carbohydrates if you are eating your soup before 6pm and a delicious topping to ensure that every bowl offers variety, taste and nutritional greatness!

Soup Base

Ingredients

2 tbsp olive oil
2 finely chopped onions
2 cloves garlic, crushed (optional)
2 celery sticks, chopped (include leaves)
2 leeks, roughly chopped
2 carrots, scrubbed and chopped
1 bay leaf
1 bouquet garni
A few grindings of black pepper
A large glass of dry white wine, dry sherry or fresh apple juice/water mixed
2 pints stock - homemade vegetable or chicken or *Kallo Very Low Salt* cubes

Seasonings

Sea salt crystals or low sodium salt (*Solo* salt is a *good choice*)
Herbamare (regular or spicy)
Miso paste
Dried herbs (parsley, thyme, rosemary, oregano, mint etc. or mixed herbs)
Spices (cumin, ginger, nutmeg, turmeric, paprika, curry etc)
Spice mixes and pastes (Thai, Greek, Cajun, garam masala etc)
Mustard powder
Lemon or orange juice
Runny honey
Anchovy essence
Tomato puree

Toppings

A spoonful of pesto
A spoonful of live natural yoghurt or tzatziki
A spoonful of salsa
A swirl of nut or seed oil
A swirl of seasoned olive oil (chilli, basil etc)
A handful of bean sprouts
A handful of toasted nuts and/or seeds
Chopped fresh herbs

Method

1. Warm the olive oil in a large pan.
2. Add the onions and sauté slowly until they are golden - don't let them burn.
3. Add the garlic and sauté for another 5 minutes.
4. Add the chopped vegetables, the bay leaves, the bouquet garni and the ground black pepper and stir well.
5. Add the white wine/sherry or apple juice/water.
6. Mix the whole lot well then cover with a couple of pieces of greaseproof paper that you have soaked with cold water – make sure you fit it snugly around the edges, then put the lid on the pot and leave to simmer on the lowest possible heat. Check after 40 minutes and if they are not cooked through give them another 10/15 minutes.
7. When they are cooked but not soggy add the stock and heat through without boiling.

Options

1. Strain the stock and discard the vegetables and herbs for a clear tasty broth base.
2. Remove the bay leaf and bouquet garni and blitz/liquidise your stock for a thicker, creamier soup base (add more stock or water to thin it down if desired).
3. Remove the bay leaf and bouquet garni and use the stock as a base for a chunkier soup.
4. You can divide your clear broth or liquidised base into smaller portions in airtight containers at this stage and refrigerate for up to 2 days or freeze for future use.

Additions

- **Lean protein of choice** - cooked chicken, turkey, beef, lamb or game, fish and shellfish, tofu.
- **Fresh vegetables of choice** - green beans, spinach, courgettes, lettuce, cabbage, sprouts, mushrooms, peppers, tomatoes etc. These can be sliced, diced, shredded, ribboned or left whole. Add them to the soup base according to how long they take to cook – denser vegetables first, leafy ones last.
- **Starchy carbohydrate of choice** – tinned beans, chickpeas or lentils (drained), cooked rice, noodles or pasta, cooked barley, pumpkin or squash, sweet potato, sweetcorn and peas.

Quick Oriental Soup

Ingredients

4 shallots, unpeeled and halved
1 clove garlic peeled and left whole
3 star anise
1 red chilli, deseeded and halved
3 kaffir lime leaves
2 stalks lemongrass, bashed
1 x 1" piece of fresh ginger, peeled
A handful of coriander leaves
3 pints cold water

Seasonings

Miso paste
Oriental spice mixes and pastes
Lemon or lime juice
Fish sauce (nam plah)
Oyster sauce
Soy sauce
Rice wine

Toppings

A swirl of sesame seed oil
A handful of bean sprouts
A handful of toasted nuts and/or seeds
Chopped fresh herbs
Grated fresh coconut

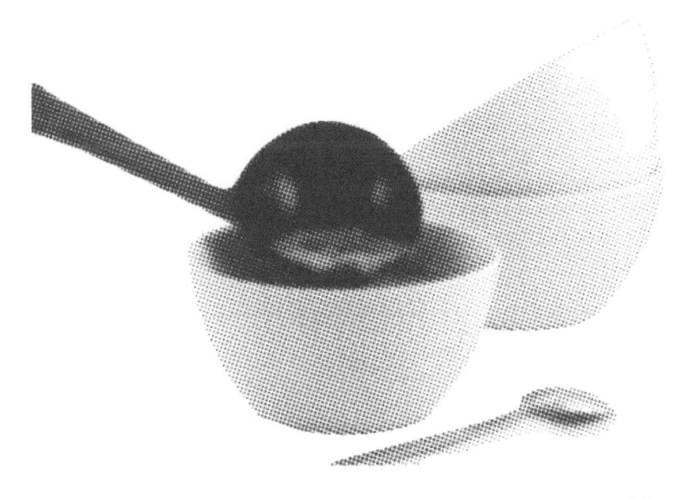

Method

1. Put all the ingredients in a large pot and cover with the water.
2. Heat through until just boiling then turn down immediately to very low and simmer for 20 to 30 minutes.
3. Strain and use immediately or refrigerate/freeze.

Additions

- **Lean protein of choice** - cooked finely sliced or shredded chicken, turkey, duck, beef or lamb, fresh fish and shellfish, tofu, whisked egg.
- **Fresh vegetables of choice** – bok choy, Chinese leaves, mustard greens, mangetout, spinach, cabbage, lettuce, cucumber, mushrooms, spring onions, seaweed, tomatoes, peppers, bean sprouts, bamboo shoots etc. These should be finely sliced, shredded or ribboned. Add them to the stock according to their cooking times – denser vegetables first, leafy ones last.
- **Starchy carbohydrate of choice** – rice vermicelli, noodles, sweet potato, sweet corn, peas.

Quick Vegetable Stock

Ingredients

1 tablespoon olive oil or rapeseed oil
1 large carrot, peeled and cut into chunks
4 sticks of celery cut into chunks
1 medium onion, peeled and cut into quarters
1 small fennel bulb, halved (optional)
2 large garlic cloves, peeled and crushed
2 pints water
1 medium tomato, halved
1 bouquet garni
1 tbsp soy sauce (optional)
1 small dried red chilli pepper (optional)
Freshly ground black pepper to taste
1 tsp sea salt flakes

Method

1. Warm the olive/rapeseed oil in a large saucepan.
2. Add the carrot, celery, onion and fennel and sauté for a few minutes until the vegetables are just beginning to soften.
3. Add the garlic and sauté for another minute.
4. Add the water, tomato, soy sauce, bouquet garni, chilli and black pepper.
5. Bring to the boil then turn the heat to low for about half an hour.
6. Strain and use immediately or refrigerate/freeze.
7. If you wish a more concentrated flavour, boil the strained stock to reduce by about a third.
8. Add the salt right at the end.

Quick Chicken Stock

Ingredients

1 tbsp olive oil
1 medium onion, finely chopped
6 skinless chicken thighs
1 litre boiling water
1 tsp sea salt flakes
1 bay leaf or 1 bouquet garni

Method

1. Warm the olive oil in a large pan.
2. Add the onions and sauté slowly until they are golden – don't let them burn.
3. Remove the onions to a bowl.
4. Brown the chicken pieces in the oil then return the onions to the pot.
5. Reduce the heat to low, cover and cook gently for 10 to 15 minutes until the chicken pieces release some of their juices.
6. Increase the heat briefly while you add the boiling water, salt and bay leaf/bouquet garni, then return to a very gentle simmer for about 20 minutes until the stock is rich and flavourful.
7. Strain and skim and use immediately or refrigerate in an airtight container for up to 2 days or freeze in small containers or ice cube trays.

Special Brown Rice

The thought of a bowl of brown rice makes many people groan, but it is quite delicious prepared this way – hot or cold!

Ingredients

1 cup organic brown rice, short or long-grained
2 cups water
½ tsp sea salt crystals
1 tbsp olive oil

Method

1. Rinse the rice well and drain it.
2. Put it in a heavy saucepan with the water, salt and olive oil.
3. Bring to the boil then cover the pot with a tight-fitting lid and reduce the heat to low.
4. Cook the rice for 45 mins, without disturbing it - if the lid is removed the steam which cooks the rice, will be lost. If you have lost track of the time and aren't sure if the rice is done, put your ear to the pot and listen (but not too close or you will burn your ear!). If there is no sound of water bubbling, the rice should be done.
5. Just before serving, fluff the grains gently with a fork.

Mejadarra with Mushrooms

Ingredients (Serves 4)

3½ oz/100g large green lentils
2 medium onions, finely chopped
1-2 tbsp olive oil
½ tsp ground turmeric
1-2 tsp freshly ground cumin seeds (already ground is fine)
1-2 tsp freshly ground coriander seeds (" " ")
½ pint 'marigold' powder stock
5½ oz/150g brown basmati rice
1 tbsp olive oil for frying mushrooms
10/12 chestnut mushrooms, sliced
Handful of fresh coriander sprigs, roughly chopped
Salt and freshly ground black pepper

Method

1. Place the lentils in a bowl and cover with cold water - soak for 2-3 hours.
2. Finely chop the onions.
3. Heat the olive oil in a pan, add the chopped onion and fry gently until softened but not browned.
4. Add the spices and stir well.
5. Drain the lentils and add to the pan with the stock. Bring to the boil, cover and simmer for about 20 mins or until the lentils are soft.
6. Meanwhile, place the rice in a small pan, cover with cold water and bring to the boil.
7. Stir once then lower the heat and cook for 3 mins.
8. Drain and rinse with cold water.
9. Stir the parboiled rice into the lentils. Add a little water to cover. Season with salt and pepper.
10. Bring to the boil, then lower the heat and cook, covered, until all the liquid is absorbed and the rice cooked.
11. Heat the remaining olive oil in a frying pan, add the mushrooms to the pan and sauté until softened and crunchy at the edges. Remove with a slotted spoon and keep warm.
12. Heat the oil left in the pan and stir fry half the chopped coriander briefly.
13. Stir the remaining coriander into the lentil mixture (mejadarra) and transfer to a warm serving dish.
14. Top with the mushrooms and stir-fried coriander and serve.

NB: you can replace the rice with bulghur wheat for a nuttier taste and if you don't like mushrooms, leave them out and top the dish with chunks of roasted aubergine and courgettes

Very Quick Mejadarra with Mushrooms

(Serves 2)

Sauté some sliced onions and sliced mixed mushrooms. Add half a tin of lentils and the same amount of cooked brown basmati rice, a teaspoon or two of powdered mixed spices (coriander, cumin, turmeric etc), cover scantily with stock made with *Marigold Swiss Vegetable Bouillon* (low salt) and simmer until the liquid more of less evaporates. Season with salt flakes and freshly ground black pepper, fluff it up with a fork and eat.

Dhal

There are loads of different ways of making this dish and recipes abound on the internet, but here's one that is particularly tasty.

Ingredients (Serves 2)

200g fresh spinach
120g tinned green or brown lentils, drained
1 medium onion, finely chopped
Olive or rapeseed oil
Small piece ginger, peeled and grated (about ½")
1 heaped teaspoon each of ground cumin, ground coriander and ground turmeric
1 garlic clove, crushed
2 tbsps natural yoghurt
Sea salt flakes and ground black pepper
¼ pint vegetable stock
2 portions quick cook brown basmati rice
A handful of fresh coriander or flat leafed parsley

Method

1. Heat a tablespoon of the oil in a pan and soften the onion and ginger for about 5 minutes.
2. Add the garlic and spices and cook for another minute, stirring.
3. Add the lentils, cover with the vegetable stock and cook slowly for 15-20 minutes (add water if it begins to look a little dry).
4. Steam the spinach, drain and chop and add to the pan.
5. Add the yoghurt then season to taste and heat through VERY slowly so the yoghurt doesn't split.
6. Serve with the cooked rice and scatter freshly chopped coriander/ parsley on top.

Lamb Tagine

Ingredients (Serves 6)

2 lb lean lamb, cut from the leg or neck fillet, cubed
1 onion, finely chopped
2-3 tbsp oil
¼ tsp saffron
¼ tsp ground ginger
½ tsp ground coriander
1 tsp ground cinnamon

Salt and black pepper
4 oz ready to eat prunes, pitted
2 tbsp honey and/or 1 tsp orange flower water, to taste
Toasted sesame seeds

Method

1. Put the meat in a large saucepan, just cover with water or stock and add the onion, oil, ginger, saffron, if used, salt and pepper to taste, coriander and cinnamon.
2. Bring to the boil, cover the pan and simmer very gently until the meat is tender and the liquid has become a rich sauce - about 2 hours.
3. Cool and freeze at this stage if desired.
4. Add the prunes and simmer for 20 minutes longer.
5. Stir in the honey or orange flower water and cook for a further 15 minutes, uncovered if necessary to concentrate the sauce.
6. Taste for seasoning, grind on fresh pepper and sprinkle with orange flower water.
7. Garnish with toasted sesame seeds.

Special Porridge

Ingredients (Serves 2)

120g porridge oats
840 ml water

Method

1. Mix the oats with half the water and leave to soak if you have time (overnight is good if you remember).
2. Add the remaining water and stir thoroughly.
3. Put on a medium heat in a good thick-based pan and bring to the boil, stirring continuously.
4. Reduce the heat and simmer for 6 minutes, stirring occasionally.
5. Serve in warmed bowls and top with some of the following:-

Toppings

A dollop of Greek yoghurt and a drizzle of runny honey
A handful of mixed berries and a scatter of toasted flaked almonds
Half an apple sliced and a dusting of cinnamon
Sliced banana and mixed seeds
A spoonful of Manuka honey stirred in
Mango slices and mixed spice
Mixed nuts, seeds and dried fruit

Cold Oats

Ingredients (Serves 1)

A couple of handfuls of raw oats
A handful of mixed nuts, seeds and dried fruit of choice
Fresh apple or pineapple juice
A tablespoon of natural live yoghurt
Fresh fruit of choice
Ground cinnamon or nutmeg

Method

1. Put the oats and the mixed nuts, seeds and dried fruits in a bowl and cover with the apple or pineapple juice.
2. Leave to soak overnight or as long as you can to soften the oats, plump up the dried fruits and make the nuts and seeds more digestible.
3. Top with the yoghurt and fresh fruit and sprinkle with the ground cinnamon or nutmeg.

More ways with oats

Porridge Smoothie

A hot smoothie for a cold morning

Ingredients (Serves 1)

25g porridge oats
300ml skimmed milk or soya milk
100g natural yoghurt
50g blueberries
50g strawberries

Method

1. Place the oats and milk in a small saucepan and simmer for 2 minutes.
2. Pour the mixture into a food processor/liquidiser with the remaining ingredients.
3. Blend until smooth.
4. Water down with a little hot water if it is too thick.
5. Sprinkle some toasted flaked almonds on top for extra crunch.
6. Serve with a spoon.

Honeyed Muesli

Ingredients (Serves 1)

100g porridge oats
20g each of almonds, hazelnuts and walnuts
2 tbsp sunflower seeds
1 tbsp clear honey
30g dried apricots, chopped
200g mixed berries
Tablespoon water

Method

1. Preheat the oven to 200C/Gas Mark 6.
2. Mix the oats, nuts and seeds with the honey in a bowl then transfer to a baking/roasting tin.
3. Spread the mixture evenly over the tin.
4. Bake for 5 minutes or until toasted.
5. Allow to cool.
6. Place the fruit in a pan with the water and cook slowly until soft.
7. Spoon over the muesli and serve.

Quick Fishcakes

Ingredients (Makes 4 fishcakes)

400g tinned salmon, sardines or other oily fish
85g oats
80ml skimmed milk
1 egg
2 tbsp chopped fresh herbs of choice
Olive or rapeseed oil
Sea salt flakes and freshly ground black pepper
Wholemeal breadcrumbs (about 5 or 6 tbsps)
Tzatziki or raita to serve

Method

1. Mix all the tinned fish, oats, milk, egg and herbs together.
2. Add a pinch or two of salt flakes and a few grindings of black pepper.
3. Divide the mixture into 4 and shape into fishcakes.
4. Cover completely with the breadcrumbs and chill for 20-30 minutes.
5. Heat a little oil in a frying pan over a medium heat until hot but not smoking.
6. Brown the fishcakes for about 3 minutes on each side.
7. Serve with a good dollop of tzatziki or raita.

You can also coat whole fresh fish or fish fillets in oats mixed with a little salt and pepper before baking, mix oats with a little honey and top stewed fruit for a healthy crumble, use a mixture of oats and other cereal grains mixed with dried fruit, nuts, seeds and honey or maple syrup to make your own flapjacks and cookies or make healthy, filling muffins. They are a great addition to a morning or lunchtime smoothie or use oat milk (Oatly is widely available) instead of other milks in your smoothies or on your morning cereal.

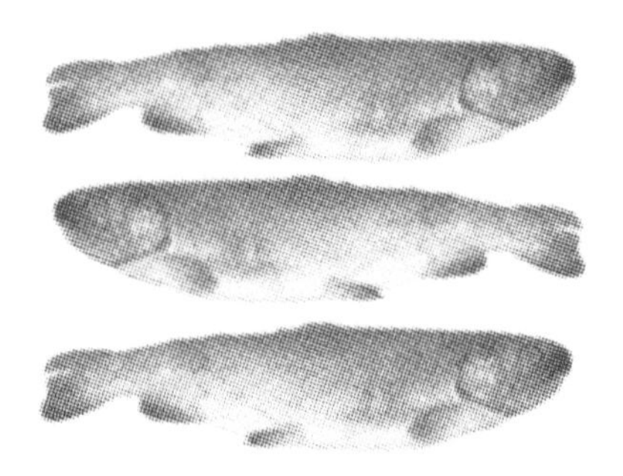

Prawn, Lemon, Basil + Spring Onion Risotto

Ingredients (Serves 2)

Olive oil
½ onion, finely chopped
1 clove of garlic, peeled and finely chopped
150g risotto rice
75ml white wine
750ml warm light vegetable stock
A bunch of spring onions, thinly sliced
150g cooked peeled prawns
3 tablespoons low-fat crème fraîche
A squeeze of lemon
½ bunch of basil, chopped
Salt and freshly ground black pepper

Method

1. Heat up a splash of oil and gently fry the onion and garlic until translucent. Add the rice and continue frying for two minutes. Add the wine and continue stirring until the wine is absorbed.
2. Now start to add the stock, ladle by ladle, stirring until the stock is absorbed between each spoonful.
3. Give the risotto lots of tender loving care, by stirring regularly, and the creamy starch will come out of each grain. Continue like this for 10 to 15 minutes.
4. Add the spring onion to the risotto, continue cooking for five minutes and then add the prawns and crème fraîche.
5. Now this is the important point. You need the rice to be *al dente*, (which means firm-to-bite, not soft and overcooked), so keep tasting it until it is time to take it off the heat (it will probably need another five minutes).
6. Add a squeeze of lemon and stir through the basil. Check the seasoning and then, for the final touch, grate some lemon zest over the top.

Try crab or chicken instead of the prawns, or replace the basil with chives or tarragon.

Baked Asparagus + Ham Risotto

Ingredients (serves 4)

2 pints chicken stock
1 tbsp olive oil
1 onion, finely chopped
1 ½ cups arborio rice
1 bunch asparagus, trimmed, cut into 3cm lengths
Couple of handfuls of frozen peas
2 tbsps grated parmesan cheese
150g sliced ham

Method

1. Preheat oven to 170°C. Bring stock to the boil in a saucepan over high heat. Reduce heat to low and simmer.
2. Meanwhile, heat a large flameproof casserole over medium heat. Add onion. Cook, stirring, for 5 minutes or until onion is soft. Add rice. Stir to coat.
3. Add stock to rice. Stir to combine. Transfer dish to oven. Bake, covered, for 30 minutes or until rice is just tender and stock is nearly all absorbed.
4. Meanwhile, steam asparagus and peas for 2/3 minutes then drain.
5. Add parmesan, asparagus, peas and ham to risotto. Stir to combine. Season with pepper. Serve.

Essential Smoothie

Filling, fat burning and exploding with antioxidants.

Ingredients (Serves 2)

2 tablespoons mixed raw seeds (pumpkin, sunflower, flax etc)
3 ice cubes
200g mixed red/purple berries (raspberries, blueberries, blackcurrants, brambles strawberries, stoned cherries etc)
100g watermelon, seeds included
200g silken tofu, drained and sliced
¾ litre rice milk or skimmed milk

Method

1. Place the seeds in a food processor/liquidiser and grind until pulverised (if your processor is not strong enough use a coffee grinder then transfer to the blender).
2. Add the ice cubes and the rest of the ingredients and run on full power until smooth and creamy.
3. Transfer to a tall glass and sip slowly.

Part 3. Chapter Twenty

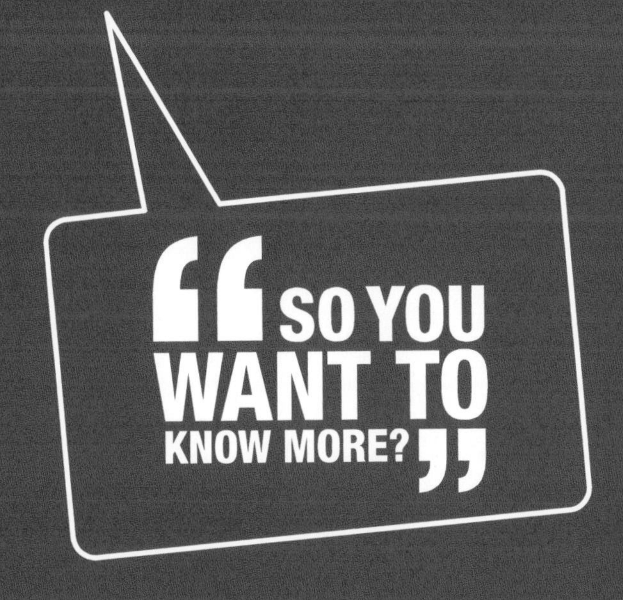

If you've got room for dessert, go for it!

Books to Browse

Health Defence by Dr Paul Clayton ISBN 0905553632

Fats that Heal Fats that Kill by Udo Erasmus ISBN 0920470386

Biochemical Individuality by Roger J Williams ISBN 0879838930

Thirst by Nigel Slater ISBN 1841157686

Super Juice by Michael Van Straten ISBN 1840001488

The Greens Cook Book by Deborah Madison ISBN 0-553-50524-6

Wagamama Cookbook by Hugo Arnold ISBN 1856266494

New Covent Garden Soup Co. Book of Soups ISBN 075220503X

Websites to Surf

To find a recognised Nutritional Therapist in your area:

The British Association for Applied Nutrition and Nutritional Therapy
BANT members are qualified in both the science of nutrition and clinical practice.

www.bant.org.uk.

The Institute for Optimum Nutrition
All listed nutritional therapists hold the DipION Diploma and are registered with BANT.

www.ion.ac.uk.

Detox Retreats:

Detox International
Offer 7 day holistic detox retreats in Spain and Portugal.

www.detox-international.com

Diets Delivered to your Door:

Pure Package
Freshly prepared, ethically sourced and convenient meals delivered daily.

www.purepackage.com

Boot Camps:

The New You Boot Camp

www.newyoubootcamp.com

The Ultimate Boot Camp

www.ultimatebootcamp.com

Supplements:

Positive Health Shop
Offers a wide range of quality supplements and nutritional advice.

www.positivehealthshop.com

Research Sources to Study

The Cochrane Library
Contains high-quality, independent evidence from systematic reviews, clinical trials and medical research studies.

www.thecochranelibrary.com

Natural Medicines Comprehensive Database
Provides evidence-based clinical information on natural medicines.

www.naturaldatabase.com

Food Products to Try

Hale & Hearty
A range of wheat-free and gluten-free products available from Sainsbury's, Tesco, Waitrose and independent food retailers.

www.halenhearty.co.uk

Olly Oils
An excellent range of delicious, cold pressed, unrefined oils for cooking and dressing (olive, avocado, flaxseed, rapeseed, safflower, macadamia, sesame) which are available from selected stores and online.

www.ollyoils.com

Clearspring
Award winning supplier of organic and traditional foods (teas, sauces, oils, pastas, nut and seed butters etc) available from supermarkets and independent food retailers.
www.clearspring.co.uk

Shops to Visit

National Association of Health Stores
Search for your local health store and experiment with a great selection of natural and organic foods. The staff are well-trained in most cases and can advise on the suitability of products.

www.nahs.co.uk

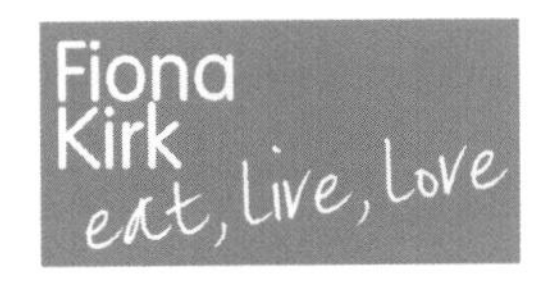

For more information visit
www.fionakirk.com

Glossary of Terms

A

Absorption: the process by which nutrients are taken from the intestines into the bloodstream then into body cells.

Acidic: having a pH of less than 7.

Adrenaline: a hormone that is produced by the adrenal gland when stress or danger is sensed by the body. It increases blood pressure, heart rate and blood flow to muscles.

Aerobic: requiring oxygen.

Alkaline: having a pH of more than 7.

Amino Acids: the basic building blocks from which proteins are assembled. There are eight essential amino acids which must be derived from the protein foods we eat to enable the body to rebuild and repair.

Anaerobic: the absence of oxygen or the absence of a need for oxygen.

Anorectics: drugs marketed as appetite suppressants.

Antibody: a type of protein produced by the body's immune system when harmful substances (antigens) are detected. Each type of antibody is unique and defends the body against one specific type of antigen.

Antioxidants: dietary substances capable of neutralising free radicals which in excess, could otherwise cause damage to body tissue and lead to cell dysfunction.

B

Bile: a yellow/green fluid made in the liver and stored in the gallbladder which passes into the small intestine where some of its components aid in the digestion of fat.

Body Mass Index (BMI): a measure of body fat.

Basal Metabolic Rate (BMR): The metabolic rate as measured under basal conditions, 12 hours after eating, after a restful sleep, no exercise or activity preceding test, elimination of emotional excitement and occurring in a comfortable temperature.

C

Calorie: a unit of measurement of energy. One calorie is defined as the amount of energy required to raise one cubic centimetre of water by one degree centigrade.

Carcinogens: cancer-causing agents.

Cardiovascular: referring to the heart and blood vessels.

Cell Membrane: the barrier that separates the contents of a body cell from its outside environment and controls what moves in and out of the cell.

Coenzyme: a molecule that binds to an enzyme and is essential for its activity, but is not permanently altered by the reaction. Many coenzymes are derived from vitamins.

Cofactor: a compound that is essential for the activity of an enzyme.

Colon: the portion of the large intestine that extends from the end of the small intestine to the rectum. The colon removes water from digested food after it has passed through the small intestine and stores the remaining stool until it can be evacuated.

D

Detoxification: the process of getting rid of toxic matter from the body.

Diabetes Mellitus: a chronic metabolic disease, characterised by abnormally high blood glucose (sugar) levels, resulting from the inability of the body to produce or respond to insulin.

Diuretic: an agent that increases the formation of urine by the kidneys, resulting in water loss.

DNA: the genetic coding found in the nucleus (the brain) of every body cell which determines specific characteristics and functions within the body.

E

Electron: a stable atomic particle with a negative charge.

Enzymes: made up of a complex of amino acids, enzymes are part of every chemical reaction in living things. These include all digestion, growth and building of cells, any breakdown of substances such as vitamins and nutrients and all reactions involving the transformation of energy.

Essential Fatty Acids: linoleic acid (Omega 6s) and linolenic acid (Omega 3s) are 'essential' because the body cannot make them or work without them. They are important for brain development, controlling inflammation, blood clotting, heart health etc and must be derived from our diet.

F

Fermentation: an anaerobic process that involves the breakdown of dietary components to yield energy.

Free Radicals: highly reactive molecules possessing unpaired electrons that are produced during the metabolism of food and energy. They are believed to contribute to the molecular damage and death of vital body cells and may be a factor in ageing and disease. Antioxidants help neutralise them.

G

Gene: a region of DNA that controls a specific hereditary characteristic, usually corresponding to a single protein.

Glucagon: a hormone responsible for helping maintain balanced blood sugar levels. When blood sugar levels get too low, glucagon activates glucose production in the liver, as well as regulating the release of glycogen from muscle cells.

Glucose: a 6-carbon sugar which plays a major role in the generation of energy for living organisms.

Glycaemic Index (GI): an index of the blood glucose-raising potential of the carbohydrate in different foods. The GI is calculated as the area under the blood glucose curve after a test food is eaten, divided by the corresponding area after a control food (glucose or white bread) is eaten. The value is multiplied by 100 to represent a percentage of the control food.

Glycaemic Load (GL): an index that simultaneously describes the blood glucose-raising potential of the carbohydrate in a food and the quantity of carbohydrate in a food. The GL of a food is calculated by multiplying the GI by the amount of carbohydrate in grams provided by a food and dividing the total by 100.

Glycogen: a large chain of glucose molecules used to store energy in cells, especially muscle and liver cells.

H

Hormone: a chemical, released by a gland or a tissue, which affects or regulates the activity of specific cells or organs. Complex bodily functions, such as growth and sexual development are regulated by hormones.

I

Immune System: the body's defence against infectious organisms and other invaders. Through a series of steps called the immune response, the immune system attacks organisms and substances that invade body systems and cause disease.

Insulin: a hormone secreted by the beta-cells of the pancreas required for normal glucose metabolism.

L

Laxative: a food, compound or medication which, when consumed either induces bowel movements or loosens the stool.

M

Macronutrient: nutrients required in relatively large amounts; macronutrients include carbohydrates, protein and fats.

Malabsorption: poor absorption of nutrients from food.

Metabolism: the sum of the processes (reactions) by which a substance is taken in and incorporated into the body or detoxified and excreted from the body.

Micronutrient: a nutrient required by the body in small amounts, such as a vitamins and minerals.

Minerals: nutritionally important elements which are composed of only one kind of atom. They are inorganic (do not contain carbon as do vitamins and other organic compounds).

Monounsaturated fats: fatty acids with only one double bond between carbon atoms.

Mucous Membranes: the moist, inner lining of some organs and body cavities (nose, mouth, lungs, stomach etc). Glands in the mucous membranes make mucus, a thick, slippery fluid.

N

Neurotransmitter: a chemical that is released from a nerve cell and results in the transmission of an impulse to another nerve cell or organ. Dopamine and serotonin are neurotransmitters.

Nutrient: any substance that can be metabolised by a living creature to provide energy and build tissue.

O

Omega 3's: see 'Essential Fatty Acids'.

Omega 6's: see 'Essential Fatty Acids'.

Optimum Health: in addition to freedom from disease, the ability of an individual to function physically and mentally at his/her best.

Oxidation: a chemical reaction that removes electrons from an atom or molecule.

Oxidative Damage: damage to cells caused by free radicals.

P

Palaeolithic Diet: prehistoric diet and lifestyle.

Pancreas: a small organ located behind the stomach and connected to the small intestine. The pancreas synthesises enzymes that help digest food in the small intestine and hormones, including insulin, that regulate blood glucose levels.

pH: a measure of acidity and alkalinity.

Phytonutrients: compounds derived from plants in our diet.

Placebo: an inert treatment that is given to a control group while the experimental group is given the active treatment. Placebo-controlled studies are conducted to make sure that the results are due to the experimental treatment rather than other factors associated with participating in the study

Polyunsaturated Fats: fatty acids with more than one double bond between carbons.

Protein: a complex organic molecule composed of amino acids in a specific order. The order is determined by the sequence of nucleic acids in a gene coding for the protein. Proteins are required for the structure, function and regulation of body cells, tissues and organs and each protein has unique functions.

S

Satiety: refers to the feeling of satisfaction or 'fullness' produced by the consumption of food.

Saturated Fats: fatty acids with no double bonds between carbon atoms.

Small Intestine: the part of the digestive tract that extends from the stomach to the large intestine. The small intestine includes the duodenum (closest to the stomach), the jejunum and the ileum (closest to the large intestine).

Supplement: a nutrient or phytochemical supplied in addition to that which is obtained in the diet.

T

Thermogenic: production of heat.

Thyroid: a butterfly-shaped gland in the neck that secretes thyroid hormones. Thyroid hormones regulate a number of physiologic processes, including growth, development, metabolism and reproductive function.

***Trans* fats:** hydrogenated or partially hydrogenated oils.

V

Vitamin: an organic (carbon-containing) compound necessary for normal physiological function that cannot be synthesised in adequate amounts and must therefore be obtained in the diet.

INDEX

Lightning Source UK Ltd.
Milton Keynes UK
UKIC01n2325030914
238048UK00002B/2